OBJECTS
OF
DESIRE

A showcase of modern erotic products
and the creative minds behind them

Text by Rita Catinella Orrell
Design by Jason Scuderi

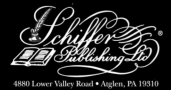

Schiffer Publishing Ltd®

4880 Lower Valley Road • Atglen, PA 19310

Designed by Jason Scuderi
Cover design by Jason Scuderi
Production design by Danielle D. Farmer
Cover photo by Michael Topolovac/Crave
Back cover photo by Rosebuds SARL
Type set in DIN
ISBN: 978-0-7643-5104-4
Printed in China

Published by Schiffer Publishing, Ltd.
4880 Lower Valley Road
Atglen, PA 19310
Phone: (610) 593-1777; Fax: (610) 593-2002
E-mail: Info@schifferbooks.com
Web: www.schifferbooks.com

For our complete selection of fine books on this and related subjects, please visit our website at www.schifferbooks.com. You may also write for a free catalog.

Schiffer Publishing's titles are available at special discounts for bulk purchases for sales promotions or premiums. Special editions, including personalized covers, corporate imprints, and excerpts, can be created in large quantities for special needs. For more information, contact the publisher.

We are always looking for people to write books on new and related subjects.
If you have an idea for a book, please contact us at proposals@schifferbooks.com.

"Take your pleasure seriously."
— Charles Eames, American designer & architect (1907–1978)

4/26/16

Dear John + Sara,
    Congrats on this exciting new
step in your life!
Best of luck in Florida!
May life bring you
everything you desire!
                    xoxo
                    Rita
                    H.

CONTENTS

FOREPLAY

As the curator of the Museum of Sex, my daily work is based in examining, contemplating, and highlighting the diverse world that is the art, artifacts, and ephemera associated with sex and sexuality. While some of these "objects of desire" are commercial products, created across the centuries, others are the secret handmade mementos of real life encounters or personal fantasies. As an anthropologist, I'm fascinated by the history and significance of these items, which in many cases do not survive the trials of time, their associations with sex often marking them in societal conflict for preservation. Yet, to me, these artifacts are some of the most illustrative and revealing of our human nature. Through examining these objects, we witness the ever-present sociological significance of sex: then, now, and into the future.

For more than a decade, I have had the privilege to explore the diversity of these treasures that encompass the historical to the functional and represent a spectrum of objectives as well as aesthetics. In 2008, with this lens as context, I curated the exhibition *Sex in Design/Design in Sex*, designed by [the multidisciplinary design firm] Pentagram. Created at a pivotal transition in sex design as a field, the exhibition focused on how the commercial sex industry was being revolutionized by high-minded design and innovation.

At the time the sex industry was undergoing a quiet yet momentous change, with sex toys and objects of pleasure moving from the underground, transforming themselves into coveted luxury objects. Once just "novelty" items, at times made from questionable materials, a trend was materializing that heralded the evolution of thoughtfully crafted objects that looked at the marketplace from a more holistic perspective. The application of a new ideology of aesthetics not only transformed the industry internally, but also dramatically transformed its consumer base.

While the artifacts on display integrated cutting-edge materials, emerging technological advances, and in some cases scientific research on pleasure, Pentagram's "intentionally austere" exhibition design was critical to the presentation as well as the topics' reception. According to James Biber, the exhibition design lead for *Sex and Design/ Design and Sex*, "this [was] the first truly uninflected look at these beautiful and occasionally quite strange objects, and they are at their best in the rather deadpan environment we created. They didn't need any help from us to look sexy."

Here, in *Objects of Desire*, I see a natural heir to the curatorial and design principles we hoped to engage with in the exhibition. While my investigation was at the nascence of this specific design revolution, in these pages we see the maturation and evolution of the sex and design field, with a highlighting of artifacts, artisans, and visionaries. With voices and objects speaking in concert with one another—illuminating the fascinating arena of design—*Objects of Desire* serves as an education to the larger design community (and world at large) about the significance of taking sex seriously. No longer just a taboo, sex has proven itself to be a necessary space of design fluency.

Sex design is no longer something to be hidden away in a designer's portfolio. Instead, as documented here, it is a craft to be celebrated. It's finally time for sex to move out of the drawer and instead find its way to the mantelpiece.

— Sarah Forbes
Curator, Museum of Sex, New York City,
and author of *Sex in the Museum:
My Unlikely Career at New York's Most
Provocative Museum*

PREFACE

When I first began my consumer product design blog *designythings* in 2011, I was taken aback by the number of sex toys and accessories being recognized by mainstream design awards around the world. One that was particularly intriguing to me was Jimmyjane's FORM collection of rechargeable vibrators. Presented on my blog under the guise of a faux *Dear Penthouse* letter, the sleek vibes were designed by Yves Béhar's renowned San Francisco-based design firm Fuseproject. Even more interesting to me than the striking product design was the discovery of a mainstream designer proudly presenting a product designed explicitly to stimulate a woman to orgasm. I knew something big was happening in the adult products industry, and it was something good.

What I didn't realize at the time was that erotic objects were in the midst of a design revolution, one that began way before E. L. James first gave readers a peek through the keyhole of Christian Grey's well-stocked playroom in her *50 Shades* trilogy. The cheaply made, sometimes even toxic novelty products once relegated to shelves in seedy XXX shops now find themselves greatly outnumbered by sleek designs made from proven or still-emerging technologies—teledildonics, app-controlled devices, and 3D-printed designs, for example—created through the same R&D processes used for high-end consumer products. These high-tech pieces are accompanied by handcrafted objects in leather, wood, and precious metals and stones that are presented and marketed like pieces of fine art. All of these objects of desire—from wooden dildos and onyx body chains to bullet vibrators that double as elegant pendants—can now be found in curated online shops and friendly, well-lit retailers that offer consumers of all spectrums of gender and sexual orientation supportive and safe environments in which to educate themselves and explore their sexuality.

The products in this book were chosen to appeal not only to lovers of good design, say the casual, curious observer, but also to those *lovers* of good design with a serious interest in acquiring these pieces. Whether they are prototypes or mass-produced, silicone or stainless steel, the products selected for this book had to share one crucial trait—functionality. They are not intended to just sit pretty in a glass vitrine—though many are, in fact, display-worthy—but have been designed specifically to stroke, spank, adorn, and otherwise interact with our bodies to produce different sensations of pleasure and pain.

Interspersed with product features, *Objects of Desire* includes interviews with sex-positive designers, bloggers, manufacturers, shop owners, and others who, through their fearless promotion of good design, help chip away at the stigma associated with enjoying products designed for sensual pleasure. In doing so, they help to empower those consumers who appreciate the main objective of these products—to bring a little more satisfaction into our lives.

— Rita Catinella Orrell

ABOUT THIS BOOK

Editorial Approach

One of our main goals was to present the product design in an open-minded, impartial, and inclusive fashion. While we did not require manufacturers to send samples in order to be included, whenever possible we tried to view the actual products. To keep things streamlined, each listing includes the company name, product name, year launched to the market, material content, and company website. All materials are listed as disclosed by the manufacturer or designer and, for the most part, are the primary materials that come into direct contact with the body.

Before using any of the products in this book, first become familiar with the manufacturer's directions, safety warnings, and cleaning instructions. You can also visit the bloggers and other resources listed in the back of this book, which include helpful reviews, safety suggestions, and other advice. Two of the most important things to be aware of when choosing a sex toy are to look for nonporous materials and to make sure to use only water-based lubricants with silicone toys as silicone lubricant can break down the material.

On a final note, all interviews in this book were conducted between 2013 and 2015, and the opinions are those of the interviewees and not the author or publisher.

— Rita Catinella Orrell

Design Approach

Erotic design is a rather touchy subject—pun intended. During the process of putting this together, Rita and I would snicker at this type of wordplay as we emailed back and forth. As time passed, we began delving into the reality of what the erotic design industry means to people— whether on a purely taboo, physical, or emotional level. We gradually wiped the smirks off our faces, and in a sense, grew up.

For my part, I was initially drawn to this project out of innocent curiosity. Of course we spoke of emotional content, social innuendo, and other hyperbole, but in the end, we both came to the conclusion that this was first and foremost a design book that needed to be similar to an unbiased museum catalog. The pages represent stark white walls to display art without being hindered by peripheral minutia. We wanted the viewers' full attention as they gazed upon the flowing curves, material, structure, and overall design of the products.

Reflecting vast hours of research, Rita's text was written as short bursts packed with interesting and vital information. These condensed paragraphs were the perfect size for visual placement and enabled the product imagery to shine.

— Jason Scuderi

INTRODUCTION
SEX TOY REVOLUTIONS

Items crafted by humans for sexual purposes go way, way back. Dildos were made of stone, wood, and leather when those were state-of-the-art materials, and Cleopatra, we are told, even had a vibrator analog—bees buzzing madly in a papyrus box. Concomitantly, every new human invention has been turned to a sexual purpose, if it could be imagined to have such a use. *Homo faber* is a sexual creature as well as a creative one.

The beautiful and sexy items gracing these pages are for the most part the most modern of erotic playthings, yet some of them retain echoes of those old *olisbos* and *consolateurs* (archaic terms for dildos). Form follows function, at least most of the time. In fact, it's a fine line for sex toy designers to walk: honoring the actions and responses of the body and the long history of sexy gear, while at the same time envisioning something truly new that might work as well . . . or better. Today, materials and technological changes are revolutionizing not only what a sex toy designer designs, but also who designs sex toys. But it is not this field's first revolution.

Rubber fetishists will, I hope, forgive me for skipping right over the materials revolution that made latex condoms, not to mention dildos and shiny rubberwear, an erotic accessory. But I'd like to tip my jimmyhat first to the Industrial Revolution, which gave us a gift that, ever since the first vibrator rolled off an assembly line, has kept on giving.

The electric vibrator (and before it, steam-powered, hand-cranked, and clockwork-driven vibrators) are not just the spawn of industrial change. They are as much a gift of Western medicine as of its factories,

for vibrators were invented as a health accessory, most notoriously to treat a mysterious ailment called hysteria. Thanks to research done over a span of twenty years by the tireless historian Rachel Maines, we know that before vibrators came along, physicians who specialized in hysteria treatment used their hands to induce "hysterical paroxysms of release" in their mostly female patients. As cities, towns, and homes were wired for electricity, the vibrator became a coveted home healthcare product, and not until this handy item began to make cameo appearances in porn movies was the cat out of the bag.

In the early 1950s the medical establishment pretty much voted hysteria out of existence, but by then, the buzzy little item that we now consider an indispensible sex toy was well established; even when its social camouflage was exposed, it continued to sell.

The sex toy's next revolution had to do with product distribution. Maybe you could still get a vibrator at the drugstore (in fact, you still can find old-school massagers there today), but items that had no healthcare credibility were a different story. Where was a person to go to buy a dildo or butt plug, or something even kinkier? It turned out that new shopping opportunities were afforded by the so-called adult bookstore. Though, granted, many of these did not carry all that many books, they *did* give ample shelf space to "rubber goods"—or, as they were called when I was a youth, "marital aids." Items that had once been available only by mail order or from the trunk of a secretive traveling salesman's car could now be acquired on the same shopping trip as porn—what could be handier?

But another revolution was about to follow, because women—expert shoppers that so many of us are—tended not to favor these often testosterone-drenched emporia. They were too seedy, too sticky, and sometimes too frightening, and unaesthetic to boot. Most dildos were penis-shaped, rubbery, and dong-colored (no one should ever call that shade "flesh"). When Joani Blank, who would go on to found Good Vibrations, recommended vibrators to women in a 1970s pre-orgasmic support group, most recoiled: "I would never go into one of *those* places," they swore, and so instead Joani became one of the first three women in the world to open a sex toy store with women in mind. Choosing items to sell as much for design as for their other functions, she hired women to sell sex toys to women, and the rest is history.

Then women began to design and make the toys. Instead of a butterscotch-colored "mystery rubber" dong, craftswomen made silicone dildos in the shapes of dolphins and goddesses. Silicone itself was a materials revolution, brought to the adult toy world by disabled entrepreneur Gosnell Duncan, founder of Scorpio Productions. Gosnell had been an industrial chemist and knew silicone's body-safe and easy-to-clean properties would make for ideal sex toys.

But not every discerning shopper desired a dildo that looked like it came from a booth in a crafts fair, and gradually, sex toys' increasing acceptability and the "clean, well-lighted" nature of the new women's sex toy stores created the cultural conditions for the most recent revolution, the one that needed new technological options to really power it into the twenty-first century.

This revolution marries design with the technical savvy we've come to expect from all our little electronic friends.

It started gradually, with Candida Royalle's ergonomic shapes that followed body curves, and with small, powerful watch batteries instead of large AA and C-cells. Euro-styled vibrators (first from Fun Factory) made the leap to silicone, and soon were being powered by computer chip technology offering multi-function and pattern vibrations. The chips can even remember the pattern you like the best and serve it up to you next time you use the vibe. More and more vibrators became rechargeable, too, some of them via your laptop's USB port. OhMiBod made toys that vibrated to the music when you used them with an MP3 player or ambient sound, and later added Bluetooth- and app-control so they can be used when lovers are far apart.

Finally, designers were saying not "How big should this penis-shaped item be?" but "What kind of extraordinary erotic object can we create that's never been made before?"

Toys don't jack into our nervous systems yet, but give them time. Erotic playthings are the province of artists and inventors now, undergoing the biggest renaissance these coveted but for so long clandestine items have ever had.

— Carol Queen, PhD
Good Vibrations Staff Sexologist, curator of the Antique Vibrator Museum, and author, with Shar Rednour, of *The Sex & Pleasure Book: Good Vibrations Guide to Great Sex for Everyone*

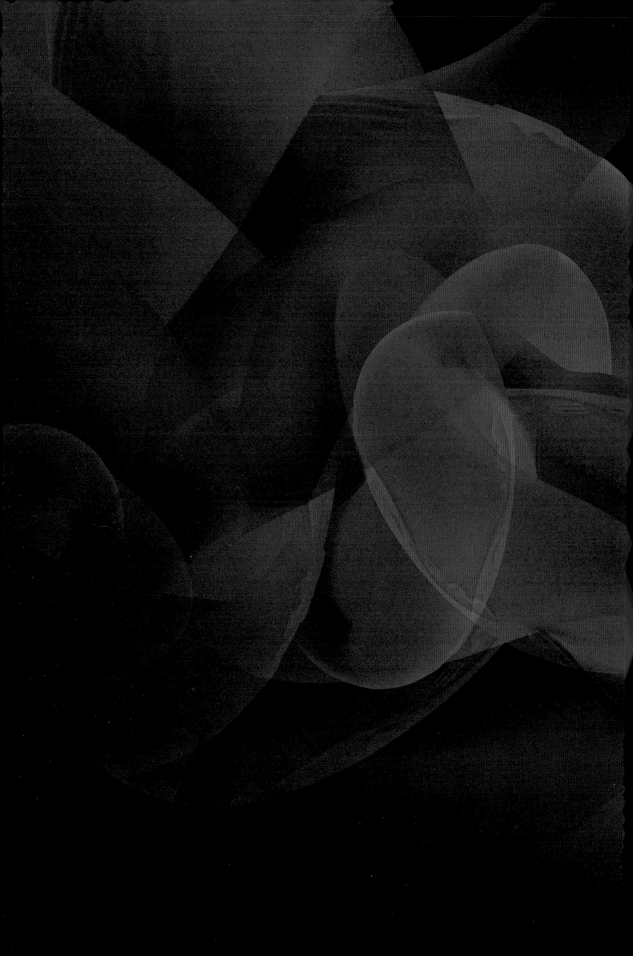

REMOTE- &
APP-CONTROLLED TOYS

WE-VIBE 4 PLUS
BY WE-VIBE

2014
Medical-grade silicone
we-vibe.com

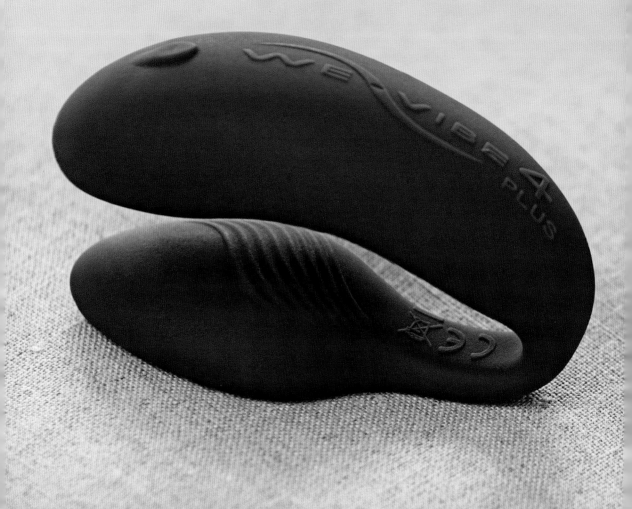

This couples vibrator is inserted into the vagina for extra stimulation to the clitoris and G-spot during intercourse. Users can independently control the intensity of the clitoral and G-spot stimulators when the vibrator is used with the We-Connect app via a private, secure connect link on their smartphone. The app also allows users to choose from ten modes and create unlimited custom playlists. Made of medical-grade silicone, the We-Vibe 4 Plus comes with a USB-powered charging base and fully charges in four hours.

LYLA 2
BY LELO

2012
FDA-approved, body-safe silicone, ABS plastic
lelo.com

LYLA 2 is a bullet-style vibrator that responds to the motion and movement of the disk-shaped remote control via LELO's SenseMotion Technology. Intended for clitoral stimulation and available with several pre-set patterns, the rechargeable, waterproof vibe is made of FDA-approved, body-safe silicone and ABS plastic.

The battery-operated remote is claimed to offer three times greater wireless range and signal strength than other wireless massagers—up to 118 feet depending on the environment. If the remote gets lost (as they often do) don't panic—the massager comes with its own multi-function control button.

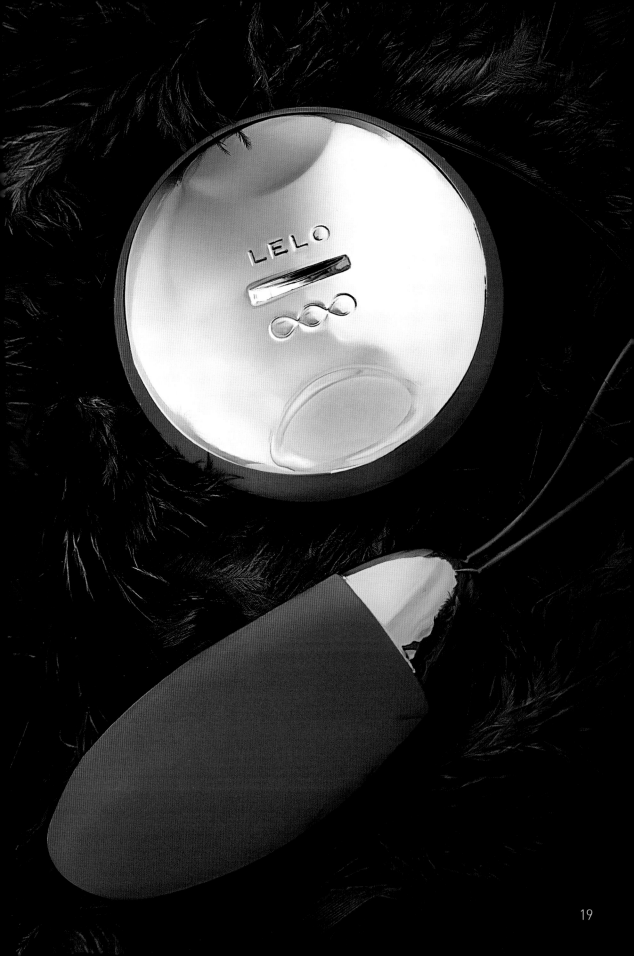

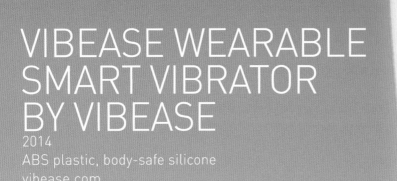

VIBEASE WEARABLE SMART VIBRATOR BY VIBEASE

2014
ABS plastic, body-safe silicone
vibease.com

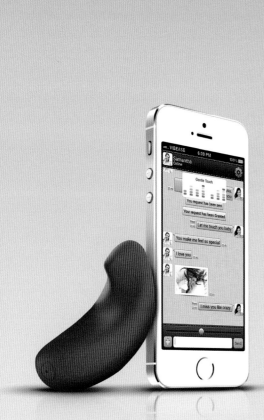

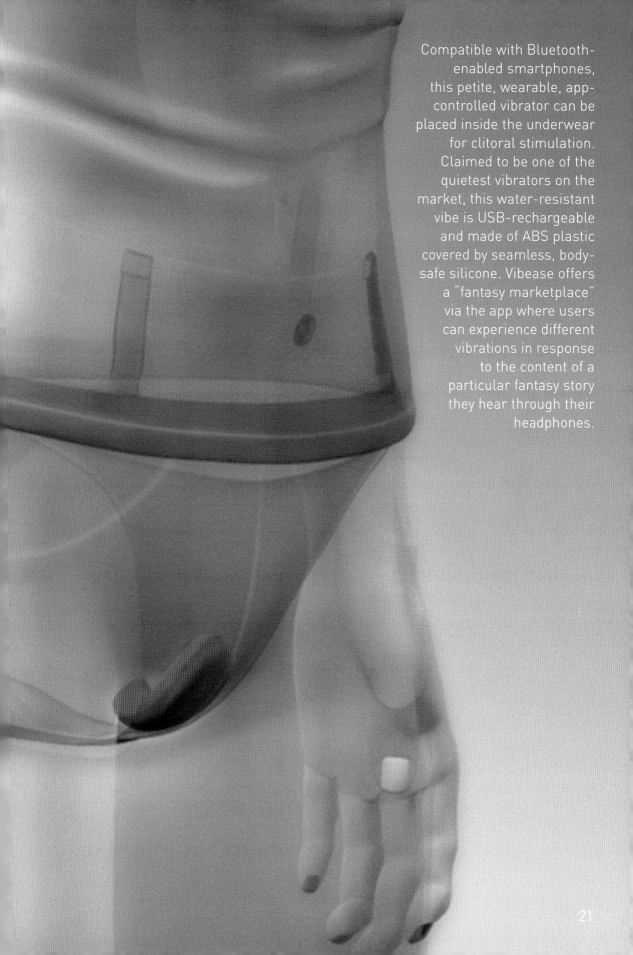

Compatible with Bluetooth-enabled smartphones, this petite, wearable, app-controlled vibrator can be placed inside the underwear for clitoral stimulation. Claimed to be one of the quietest vibrators on the market, this water-resistant vibe is USB-rechargeable and made of ABS plastic covered by seamless, body-safe silicone. Vibease offers a "fantasy marketplace" via the app where users can experience different vibrations in response to the content of a particular fantasy story they hear through their headphones.

Q&A
CLAIRE CAVANAH
AND RACHEL VENNING
FOUNDERS OF BABELAND

Are you partners in life as well as business?
No, we are and always have been pals.

What is the single most common question that customers ask you in the store about sex toys?
"How do I turn this off/on?" Seriously, though, the control buttons on vibrators aren't that obvious.) Toys for anal sex elicit a lot of questions about how to safely use them. The G-spot is also a big area for questions and fortunately there are some amazing vibrators and dildos to meet that need.

What have been the most popular toys over the years?
Well, the Magic Wand is the Cadillac of vibrators and has been on our shelves since we opened in 1993. There aren't too many toys that have that longevity, recognition, and staying power. The Rabbit Habit vibrator, made popular by the *Sex and the City* episode, captured the imagination of women everywhere and still flies out the door and is requested by name. In the past five years, the We-Vibe couples vibrator that can be worn during intercourse has been the consistent bestseller. It meets that need for vibration and clitoral stimulation during sex.

Do you feel there has been a bit of a sexual revolution for women since *Fifty Shades of Grey* or is that overstated? Has business increased since the books came out?
Fifty Shades of Grey created a sex toy frenzy! I've never seen anything like it. Customers would come in, mention the book, and either be very direct about wanting a riding crop/restraints/Ben Wa balls, or shyly ask if we had read it, too. We saw a whole new group of customers, mostly women, who had never been to a sex toy shop before and felt permission from the book's mainstream success to seek out a new experience. It was incredibly powerful to see this phenomenon and know that many people were opening themselves up to discover new pleasures.

Can you tell us a bit about your typical customer?
The majority of our customers are women in their twenties, thirties, and forties, and couples, more straight than queer.

Where are the best sex toys designed? Any favorite companies?
Right now, the Bay Area is a hotbed of sex toy innovation. Jimmyjane, Crave, and Minna Life are boutique brands based there that have been designing some of the most sophisticated and innovative toys.

Among the larger brands, LELO and Fun Factory, from Sweden and Germany, respectively, impress us with new approaches using technology that's applied to other types of products. For example, LELO has added SenseMotion remote controls to several couples toys. They operate similarly to a Wii controller and respond to motion.

OhMiBod, a US company based in Vermont, has vibes that are responsive to music and ambient sound, and also a new one that is controlled by a Bluetooth-enabled app and Skype. We-Vibe came up with the solution of adding hands-free vibration for clitoral stimulation during intercourse, and the sex toy world will never be the same.

Especially in the past ten years, we've seen amazing progress in attention to body-safe materials, quality, and technology. Our industry doesn't outcompete Apple for creating new approaches, but it's found ways to apply advances to enhance pleasure and intimacy.

As far as toy design, have you seen an improvement in the last decade? What advice would you give a young designer looking to design a sex toy?
The other thing about sex toy design that's been a delightful improvement has been the new shapes that conform more directly to a woman's body.

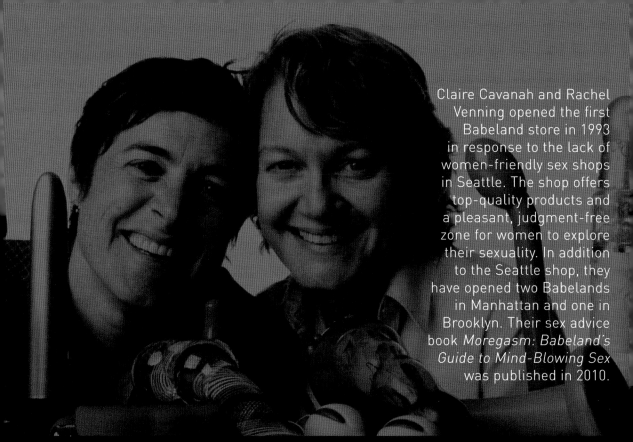

Claire Cavanah and Rachel Venning opened the first Babeland store in 1993 in response to the lack of women-friendly sex shops in Seattle. The shop offers top-quality products and a pleasant, judgment-free zone for women to explore their sexuality. In addition to the Seattle shop, they have opened two Babelands in Manhattan and one in Brooklyn. Their sex advice book *Moregasm: Babeland's Guide to Mind-Blowing Sex* was published in 2010.

The penis was definitely the model for many sex toys in the past, and we're excited to see the shift to toys that fit a woman's most sensitive parts. The Jimmyjane Form 2 is a great example. That powerful, molar-shaped little vibe just nestles right into the vulva.

Advice to a young designer? Follow your instincts. Design the toy that you want to play with and make the most of all available technologies.

Which type of toy do you feel needs the most help in the design dept? Which one do you feel is at the cutting edge?
As a category, vibrators win for cutting-edge design. In the twenty years Babeland has been selling vibrators, we have watched hard plastic Slimlines and mystery rubber vibes give way to products made of

are waterproof and rechargeable, that record the exact vibration patterns you like, in shapes that actually correspond to how bodies work. Any one of those attributes twenty years ago would have been a cause for celebration. Now we have products that do it all. Masturbation sleeves are the runner-up. Guys have never had it so good. Goodbye, pocket pussy, hello Tenga Flip!

As for needing work, I think vibrating cock rings could use a push into the twenty-first century. It's not that designers aren't applying new technologies and materials. It's more that erections are tricky. How do you affix a vibrator to something that varies so much? The materials are usually so soft that they aren't very durable, or so durable that they aren't soft enough to

There are more and more remote toys and apps on the market. What do you think about this trend towards virtual sex?
It makes sense in this era of social media and mediated socializing that sex would have its place in that trend. I don't believe sexual uses of new technology threaten real time, body-on-body sex. Whether you are separated from a lover or are lovers with someone who's not where you are, sex apps can allow you to connect and express yourself across great distances. And remote control vibes can be fun in the privacy of your home and also allow you sexual contact when you're on a date, in a club, walking down the street, at a distance of about ten feet. Technology is just the tool; it's neither good nor bad. And it can be very, very good!

BLUEMOTION
BY OHMIBOD

2014
Body-safe ABS plastic (massager),
cotton blend (panty)
ohmibod.com

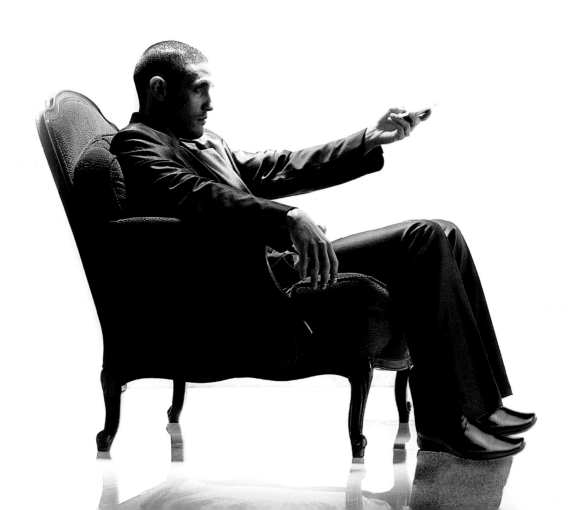

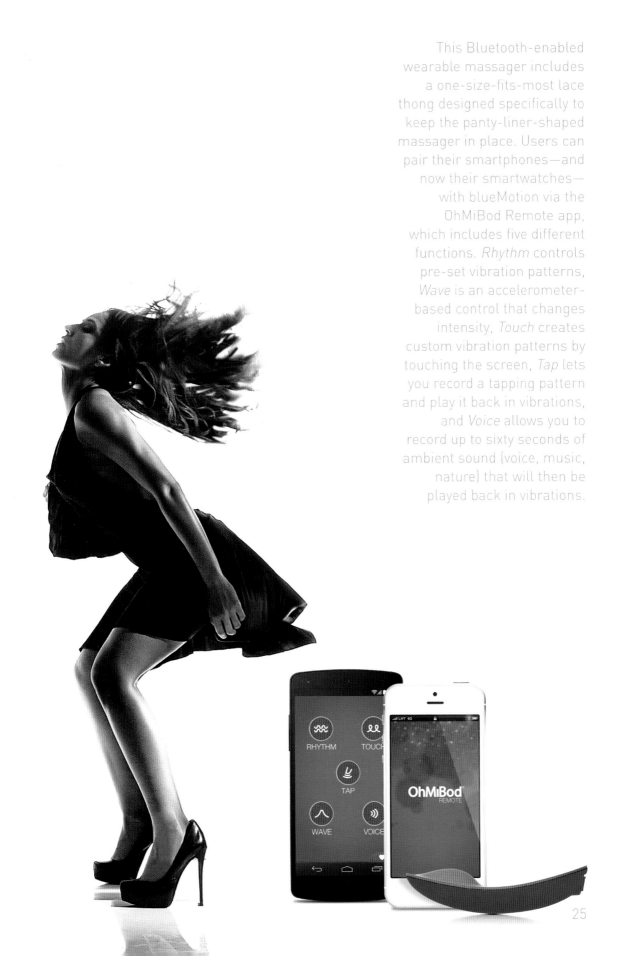

This Bluetooth-enabled wearable massager includes a one-size-fits-most lace thong designed specifically to keep the panty-liner-shaped massager in place. Users can pair their smartphones—and now their smartwatches— with blueMotion via the OhMiBod Remote app, which includes five different functions. *Rhythm* controls pre-set vibration patterns, *Wave* is an accelerometer-based control that changes intensity, *Touch* creates custom vibration patterns by touching the screen, *Tap* lets you record a tapping pattern and play it back in vibrations, and *Voice* allows you to record up to sixty seconds of ambient sound (voice, music, nature) that will then be played back in vibrations.

LOVENSE
BY HYTTO

2009 (first generation),
2011 (second generation),
2014 (third generation),
2015 (fourth generation)
Medical-grade silicone
lovense.com

Lovense is a rechargeable, teledildonic sex toy for couples looking to connect over long distances. With more than 100,000 units sold since it first launched in 2009, this interactive set of toys includes Max, a "male" masturbator sleeve, and Nora, a "female" rabbit vibrator, which use bi-directional control to respond to the movement made by each user. Advanced sensors create nearly real-time responses so that when one toy moves, the other reacts.

After the toys are synced via Bluetooth, users then "call" their partners through the Lovense smartphone app, which comes with video chat capabilities. When ready to get interactive, users simply play with the toys to send feedback to their partner. After a penis is inserted into Max, the head of Nora will start rotating—the faster Max moves up and down, the faster Nora vibrates.

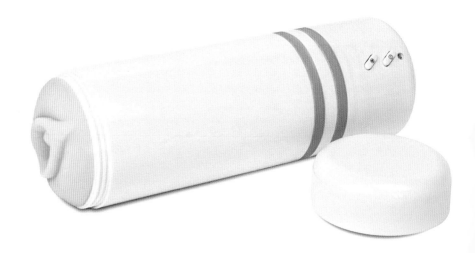

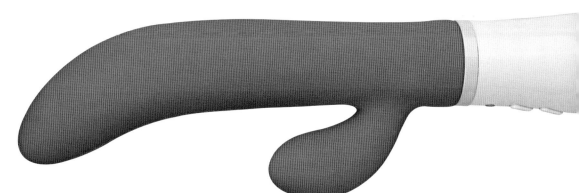

When Nora starts to move, Max's air pump will start pumping to mimic vaginal contractions; the speed of the vibration dictates the level of contractions and vibrations on the "male" end. The fun isn't limited to male/female play however; two female vibes can also respond to each other, as can two male masturbators, in the same way.

ONYX & PEARL
BY KIIROO

2015
ABS plastic,
mineral-based
elastic thermo polymer
kiiroo.com

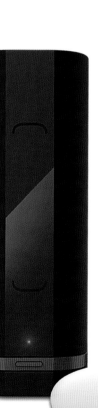

Kiiroo, a start-up tech company focusing on teledildonics, is based in Amsterdam just a stone's throw away from the city's red-light district. Partnering with male sex toy company Fleshlight, design company VanBerlo, and media company XS2, Kiiroo has developed the Pearl vibrator and Onyx masturbator, a pair of devices that communicate wirelessly worldwide. A video chat platform connects the devices via Bluetooth and can send video, audio, and tactile data to create an immersive experience. The video screen interface is even designed to appear to be a transparent piece of "glass" with translucent buttons and floating boxes to reduce distractions.

Onyx's "pleasure core" features rings that contract to mimic the movements of your partner and a Fleshlight sleeve inside. The slightly curved Pearl has five vibration modes and works both as a waterproof G-spot vibrator and as a joystick to control your partner's Onyx device through the Kiiroo platform. Although Pearl is currently a one-way device (meaning that your partner cannot control it from a distance), Kiiroo plans to expand the pairings so that Pearl can control Onyx and that two Pearls can interact together. Currently, Onyx can be controlled by either the Pearl or another Onyx device.

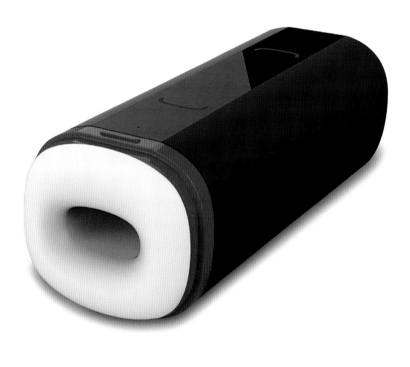

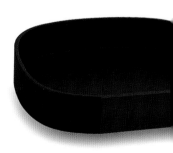

Q&A
SARAH FORBES
CURATOR OF
THE MUSEUM OF SEX

How many shows at the Museum of Sex have focused on the product design of erotic objects?
Whether it is the history of condom packaging or the visual evolution of the vibrator (which was originally created as a medical instrument), nearly all of our exhibitions touch upon the intersection of sex and design. Yet in our decade-plus of exhibition programing, our 2007 exhibition *Sex in Design/ Design in Sex* featured our most specific curatorial conversation regarding the aesthetics of commercially available erotic objects.

How has the public responded to these exhibitions?
Our *Sex in Design* exhibition was created at a very interesting time in the public acceptance of sex toys and erotic goods. For instance, many of the luxury erotic brands we are familiar with today were relatively new and did not have the widespread reach they do today. Sex objects with a refined aesthetic, rather than a "novelty" feel, were in their nascency. We exhibited these objects to specially highlight the innovation and artistry that is possible within the arena of sex.

It was truly groundbreaking to exhibit items as diverse as jade butt plugs, human hair whips, and vibrators made out of precious materials. Most of the public wasn't aware, and still to this day are not aware, these options are available in the marketplace.

Approximately how many sex toys do you have in the museum's collection? What types of toys?
The Museum of Sex has hundreds of items that could fall under the general category of "sex toys" including vibrators, cock rings, sex dolls, sex machines, and more. In collecting the artifacts, objects of art, and examples of social ephemera, many of the items in our collection cross time periods, cultures, and aesthetic traditions. Many of these artifacts often stretch the general public's perception of what a "sex toy" is thought to be.

Do you feel that the stigma related to sex toys has been improving in the last decade? Why?
Yes, tremendously. Once an object of taboo, a vibrator is said to be found in one in four households and can even be purchased in your local drugstore. I believe some of this change is due to the social relationship in regards to female sexuality. While it has been an ongoing discussion for decades, the acceptance and normalization of female sexual pleasure has increased the population of women who feel comfortable in purchasing a sex toy. It is no longer something to be purchased with embarrassment, but rather an object to be acquired with confidence, and even pride, because they are taking ownership of their own sexual satisfaction.

What are some of the latest sex toy designs or technologies that have impressed you?
I think the constant intersection of sex and technology is fascinating and what captivates me the most. Whether it is new materials or new ways to communicate, I have always seen sex designers at the forefront. Additionally, many companies are creating toys that represent larger communities and sexual interests. In addition, the trend toward personal customization is particularly exciting.

What improvements would you like to see in sex toy design?
While our bodies have certain similarities in terms of form, toys that capitalize on the fact that stimulation desires vary wildly depending on the individual and the moment in which the toy is being used are great improvements for the field. While some people are happy to purchase many sex toys, each with their particular aptitudes, many are looking for toys that can also be multi-faceted and adapt to their changing desires.

Is there one country/region that produces the most interesting sex toy designs?
I consistently see some beautiful sex-related objects coming from the UK. While this part of the world has often been associated with a more buttoned-up society, there are some stunning pieces being crafted there.

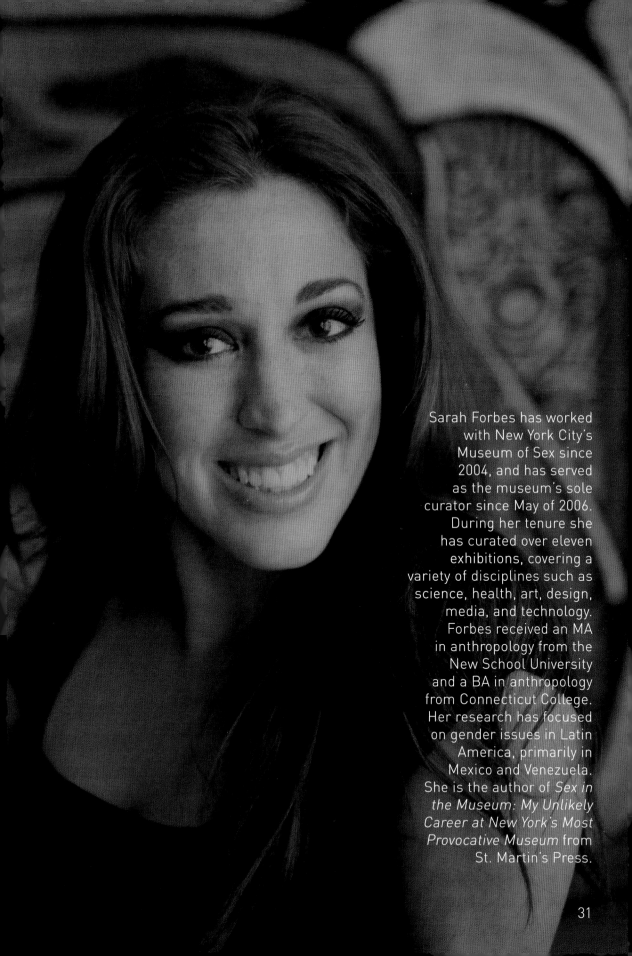

Sarah Forbes has worked with New York City's Museum of Sex since 2004, and has served as the museum's sole curator since May of 2006. During her tenure she has curated over eleven exhibitions, covering a variety of disciplines such as science, health, art, design, media, and technology. Forbes received an MA in anthropology from the New School University and a BA in anthropology from Connecticut College. Her research has focused on gender issues in Latin America, primarily in Mexico and Venezuela. She is the author of *Sex in the Museum: My Unlikely Career at New York's Most Provocative Museum* from St. Martin's Press.

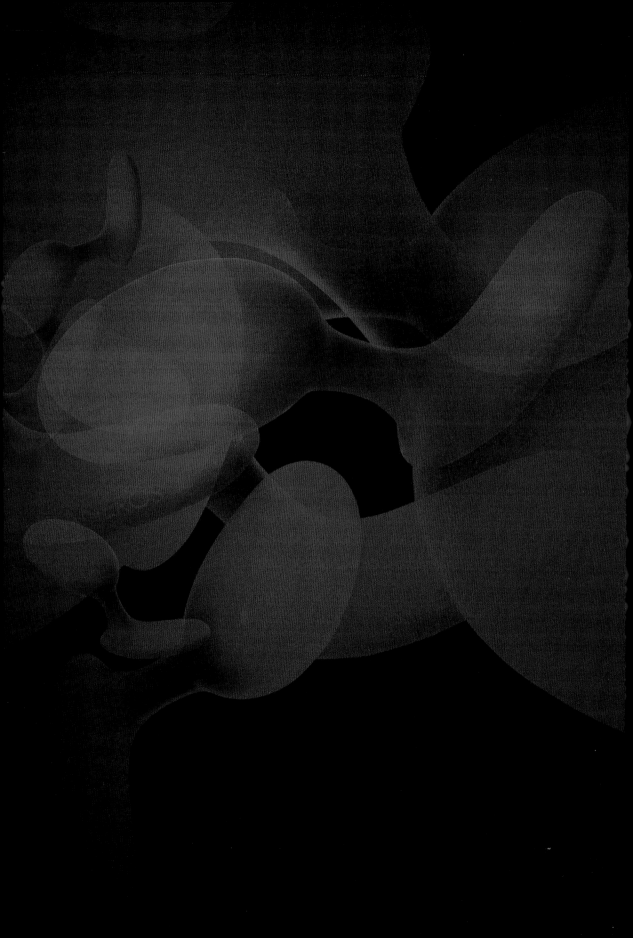

KEGEL
EXERCISERS

SINGLE & DOUBLE TRAINER TOYFRIEND BY TICKLER

2013
Body-safe silicone
ticklervibes.com

Bridging the roles of medical device and sexual aid, kegel exercisers not only help with the post-partum restoration of the pelvic muscles and prevent urine-leakage, but can also create more intense orgasms during intercourse. While women can do kegels simply by repeatedly contracting and releasing their pelvic muscles (as if to stop the flow of urine), it can be difficult to know if they are being done correctly.

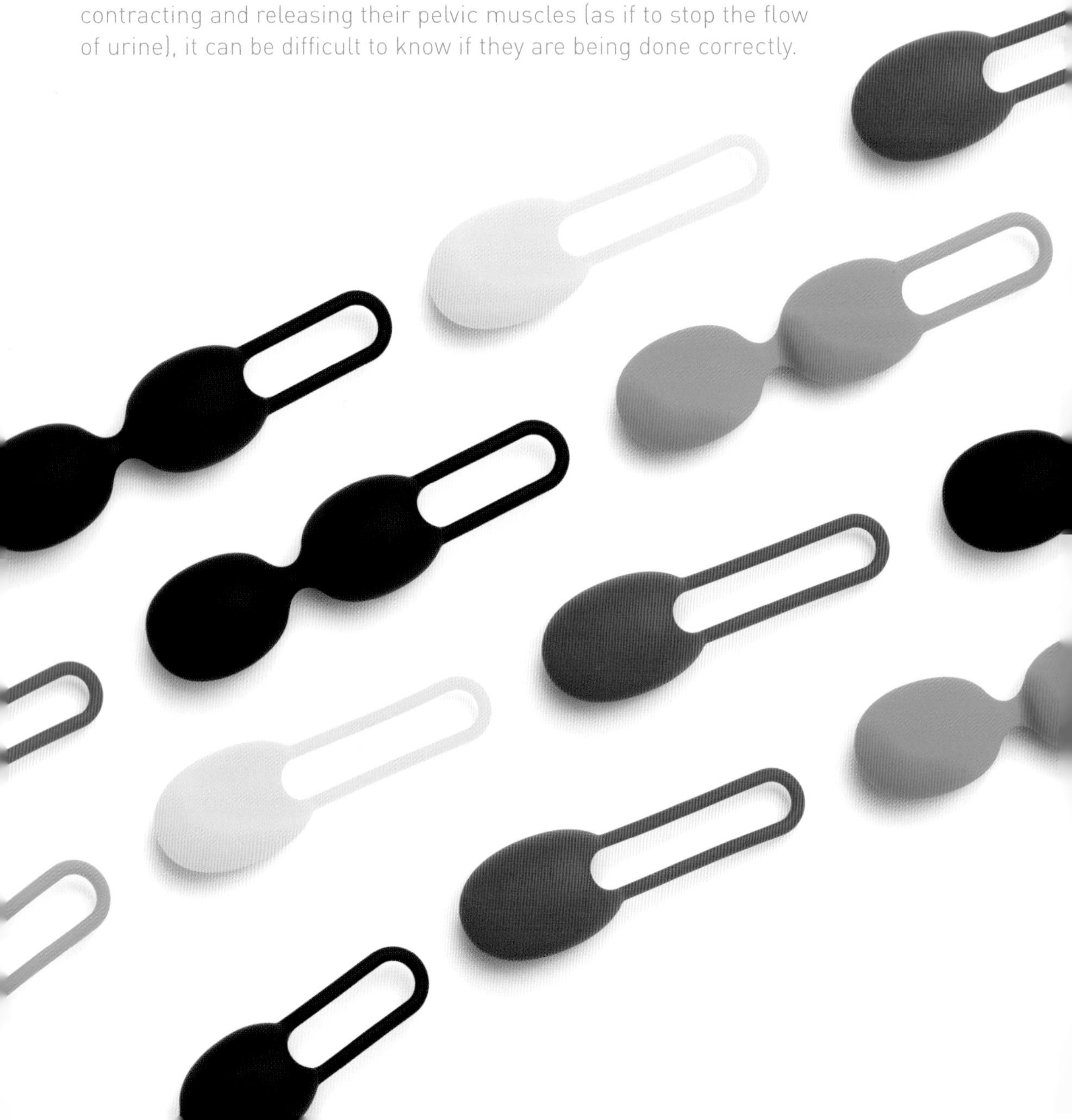

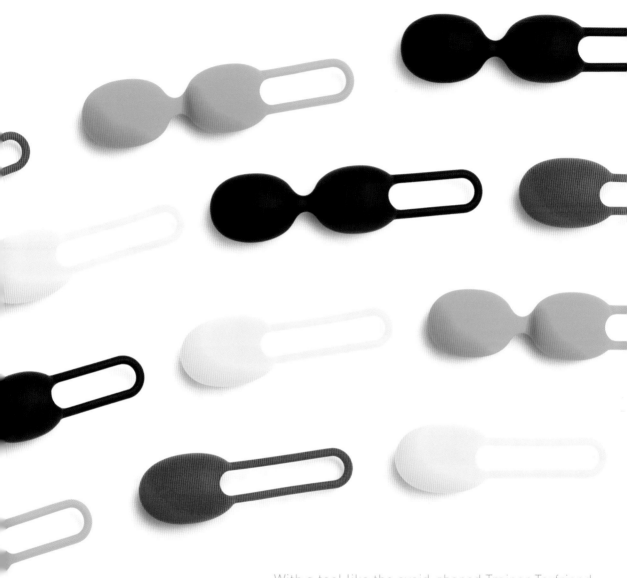

With a tool like the ovoid-shaped Trainer Toyfriend however, things become a little more obvious. Simply insert the Trainer (available in a 1.1 ounce or 2.3 ounce size) as far as it will comfortably go, and the muscles that need exercising will automatically start working once it's inside. Made out of seamless body-safe silicone in a range of cheerful colors, the Trainer just may be the easiest workout you've ever had.

LOVELIFE FLEX KEGEL WEIGHTS BY OHMIBOD

2013
Body-safe silicone
ohmibod.com

While the pink heart shapes on these kegel weights might seem cutesy to some, this PC muscle exerciser is no novelty toy. Part of the Red Dot Design Award–winning Lovelife collection from OhMiBod, Flex kegel weights are designed to accommodate everyone from first-timers to kegel pros.

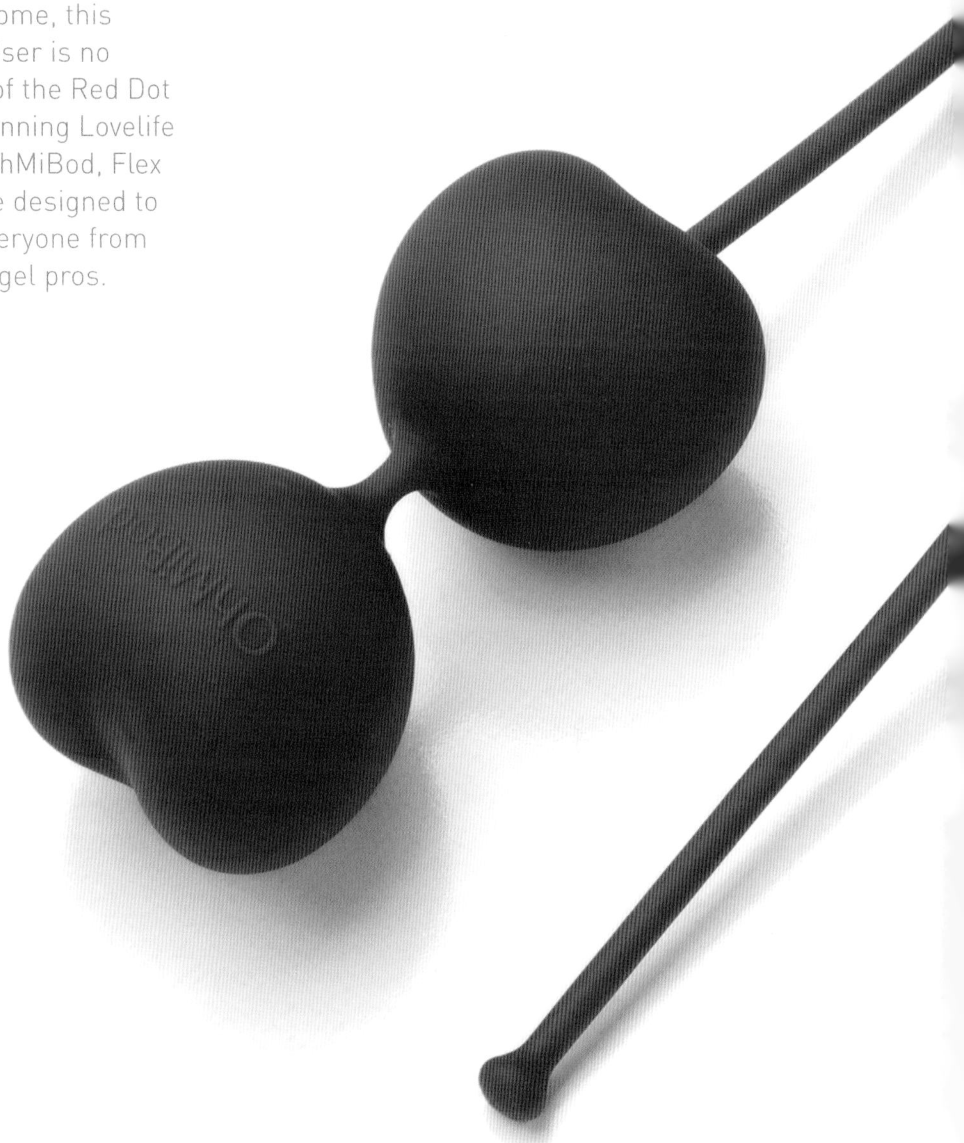

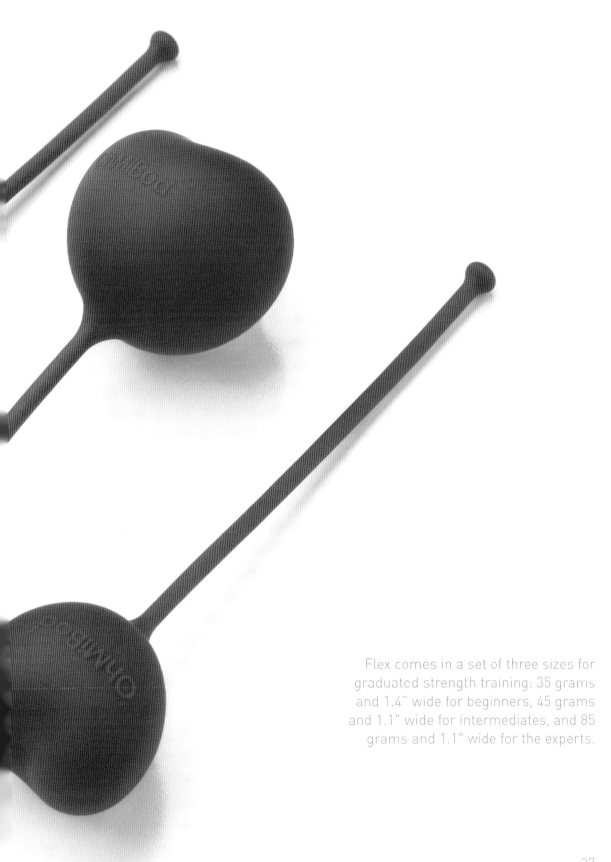

Flex comes in a set of three sizes for graduated strength training: 35 grams and 1.4" wide for beginners, 45 grams and 1.1" wide for intermediates, and 85 grams and 1.1" wide for the experts.

EVI
BY ANEROS

2012
FDA-approved, body-safe silicone
aneros.com

Evi is the first product from
the prostate stimulation
experts at Aneros to be
designed specifically for a
woman's anatomy. Primarily
intended to be used as
a kegel exerciser, the
vibration-free device offers
a hands-free experience and
can strengthen pelvic floor
muscles to achieve all of the
usual benefits: a stronger
grip during sex, enhanced
bladder control, and post-
partum recovery. Evi also
serves as a sex toy, since
the curved front of the bulb
stimulates the user's G-spot
while the handle stimulates
the clitoris. Covered in
velvet-touch silicone, Evi is
only 5.7" long and weighs
3.3 ounces, making it
discreet enough to be worn
undetectably under clothing.

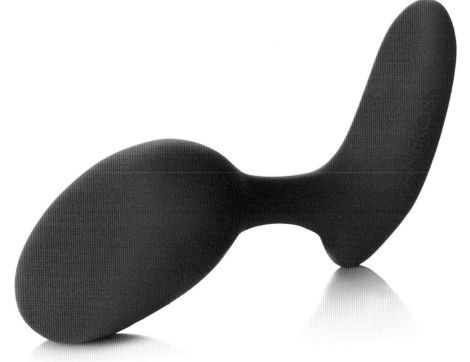

Q&A
LAUREN MARIE FLEMING
SEX BLOGGER

laurenmariefleming.com

What was the first sex toy you ever reviewed?
My very first review package came from Babeland and had the NobEssence Fling (still one of my favorite toys), the NJoy PureWand, and a Sqweel (one of my least favorite toys ever). It was quite an impressive array.

Which type of toy do you think is missing in the marketplace?
I'm not a fan of vibrators on my clit, but I like them on my nipples. I would like to see more vibrators with spacing so you could put your nipples between them.

What are the traits of a well-designed sex toy?
Simplicity. I think people are overthinking sex and overcompensating with flashy technology. That's why I love companies like Tantus and Aneros: they focus on anatomy. Good materials are a must. I don't know why we are still making and buying toxic toys, but that needs to stop.

Have you ever come across a toy that is so badly designed you won't even try it?
I've walked into stores full of toys I'd never try, mostly because their designs are novelty over function, and their materials are not ones I want to put in my body.

There seem to be more women sex toy reviewers than men sex toy reviewers. Why do you think that is?
There is sadly still a stigma against male sex toys and I think that leads to the lack of men reviewing toys. As a society, we've gotten to a point where we assume women have at least tried a sex toy in their life, but we still think the men who own them are perverts. I think this comes from the misconstrued ideas that women are difficult to get off and shouldn't just go out and have sex with people all the time, therefore they need sex toys in their lives. Whereas we believe men are easy to get off and should just go get the real thing. We also have a sad lack of trans and genderqueer people reviewing sex toys, and I'd like to see more diversity in the sex toy reviewing sphere in general.

If you could design a sex toy what would it be?
I would love something sturdy you could place any dildo in and straddle. Everything out there is so expensive or has a set cock attached to it. I want a harness on a pillow type of toy that is affordable. But other than that, I think there are brilliant minds out there making toys, so I'll stick to writing about them.

What advice would you give a young sex toy designer?
Don't overthink it. Anatomy and function beats bells and whistles any day. Apprentice with a company already doing it well, and talk to toy reviewers throughout the process. No one knows what gets people off better than we do.

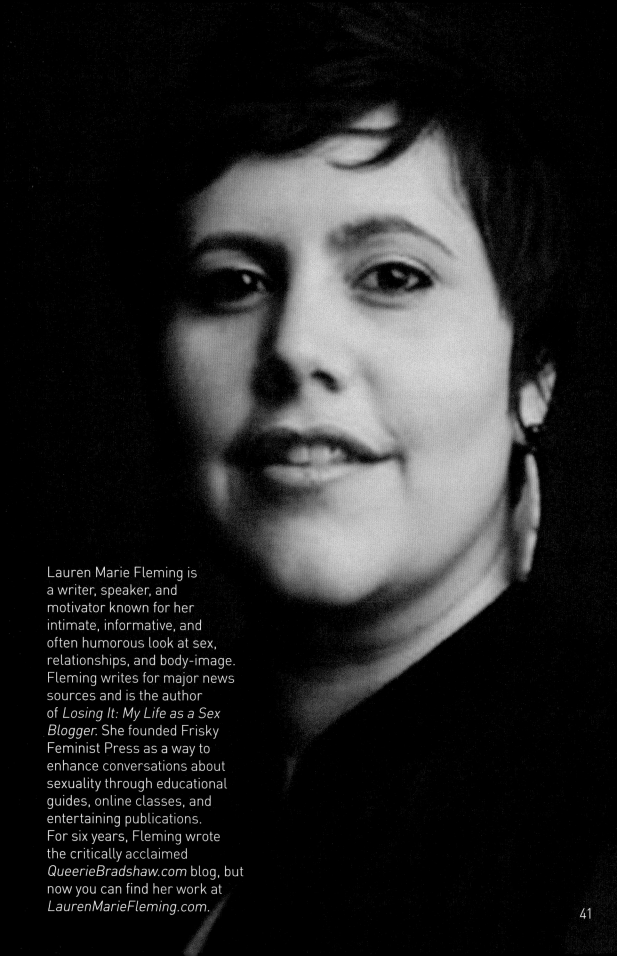

Lauren Marie Fleming is a writer, speaker, and motivator known for her intimate, informative, and often humorous look at sex, relationships, and body-image. Fleming writes for major news sources and is the author of *Losing It: My Life as a Sex Blogger.* She founded Frisky Feminist Press as a way to enhance conversations about sexuality through educational guides, online classes, and entertaining publications. For six years, Fleming wrote the critically acclaimed *QueerieBradshaw.com* blog, but now you can find her work at *LaurenMarieFleming.com.*

KGOAL
BY MINNA LIFE

2014
Medical-grade silicone
minnalife.com

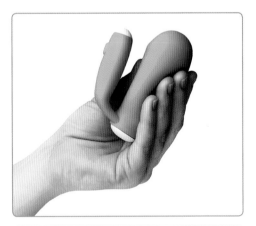

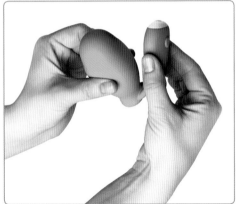

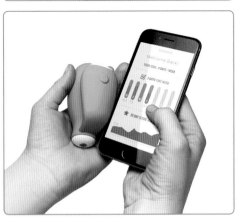

A convergence of fitness tracking and sexual health, kGoal is an interactive trainer for female pelvic floor exercise from the San Francisco-based company Minna Life. Intended to help guide pelvic floor exercise, measure performance, and track progress, the kGoal device features a squeezable pillow that is inserted into the vagina. Designed to be squishy enough to conform to a wide variety of anatomies, kGoal also has a built-in vent to allow users to optimize their fit.

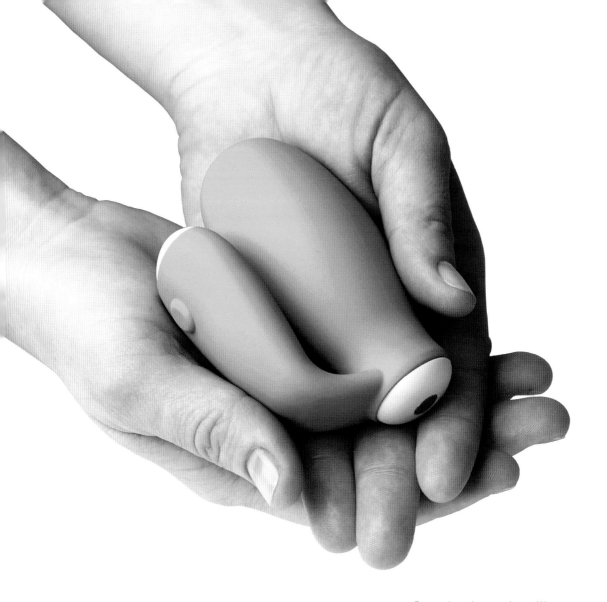

Once in place, the pillow can measure the squeezing of pelvic floor muscles, while a small motor provides real time vibrational feedback to let users know they've done the exercise right. While it's not required to use the device, the kGoal app can communicate with and control the device wirelessly, while also storing exercise history and sharing suggested workouts.

Q&A
JON MILLWARD
JOURNALIST &
IDEAS DETECTIVE

JonMillward.com/blog

Your previous studies have included deep research into the worlds of call girls, porn stars, and online dating. As an outsider to the industry, did you have the same comfort level uncovering the secrets of sex toys?
I'm very liberal and unabashed when it comes to exploring risqué topics. In fact, I find it hard to stay motivated on a project if its theme isn't at least a bit adult or potentially inflammatory. The world of sex toys was a fun one to dive into and in some ways it felt like I'd visited it before, because many of the things I'd learned in the past (from analyzing porn stars and call girls, for example) were reiterated and confirmed—mainly that human sexuality is a kaleidoscopic spectrum of interests, desires, and kinks. People are incredibly creative at coming up with ways to turn themselves and their partners on, and their creativity is reflected in the porn they watch, the call girls they (occasionally) hire, and the sex toys they buy.

What were the biggest surprises for you and for your client in the process?
I was surprised to discover that so many men, especially straight single guys, buy anal sex toys to use by themselves. I also think it's interesting that men seem to believe size matters more than women, even when buying inanimate rubber phalluses.

Women's buying habits are, in the main, less diverse than men's, mostly consisting of wearable items, vibrators, and lubricant. It's the men who branch out along the sexual adventure spectrum with wackier products, like blow-up dolls and butt plugs the size of fire extinguishers. Lovehoney was surprised to find out that 71 percent of wigs are bought by men, partly for their female partners, but also to cross-dress.

How long did it take you to analyze all 1,000,000 sex toy purchases in the study?
I spent several months on the project, about half of which was spent playing with the data, while the other half was spent creating the graphics and writing the accompanying article.

What do you attribute to the success of this particular site? Graphic design, ease of shopping? Inventory?
Lovehoney's attitude and ethos seem to be at the heart of their success: they're very relaxed, couple-focused, and no-nonsense. They have a very transparent ordering process, which starts with their site, which I think is cleanly designed and easy to navigate, on to the ordering process (which includes free delivery and returns—a huge incentive for customers!). They also have a thriving community section on their site, where thousands of men and women discuss and review their products, which of course helps give life to their brand.

Can you share any interesting customer reviews on the site that you found during your research?
Some of the product reviews are worthy of being published in a book of their own—they're absolutely fascinating and hilarious in equal measure. For instance, here's a line from a review written by a guy who had just tried out a 13.5"-long dildo for the first time and had some advice on how best to maintain it: "And every time I use it now I give it a final wash with a lemon. It seems to have calmed the smell and I can hide it now without stinking my room out." He was referring to the strong smell of the rubber.

Do you look at these types of products in a new way since the study?
I was already pretty knowledgeable about sex toys before I started this project, so nothing about the variety and types of available products surprised me. But it was nice to be able to put some hard numbers to questions about sex toy buying behavior that previously had none. Now if anybody wonders what men buy that women don't, or who buys sex swings, gimp masks, or husband voodoo dolls, they can find the answers.

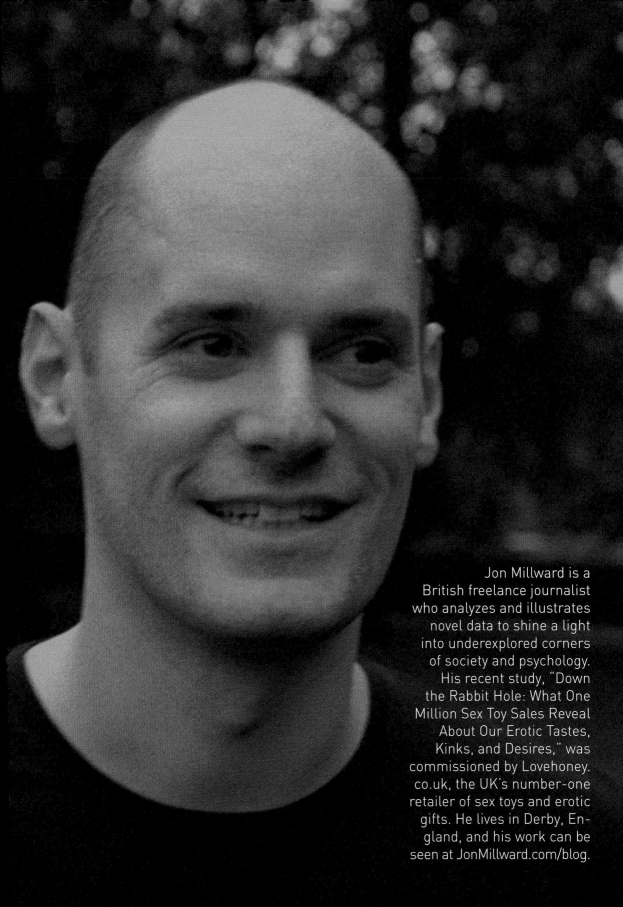

Jon Millward is a British freelance journalist who analyzes and illustrates novel data to shine a light into underexplored corners of society and psychology. His recent study, "Down the Rabbit Hole: What One Million Sex Toy Sales Reveal About Our Erotic Tastes, Kinks, and Desires," was commissioned by Lovehoney. co.uk, the UK's number-one retailer of sex toys and erotic gifts. He lives in Derby, England, and his work can be seen at JonMillward.com/blog.

SEX TOYS BY SIZE AND COLOR AND BEST-SELLING ITEMS

This spiral shows, to scale, 815 penetrative sex toys sold by Lovehoney.co.uk, the UK's biggest retailer of adult products.

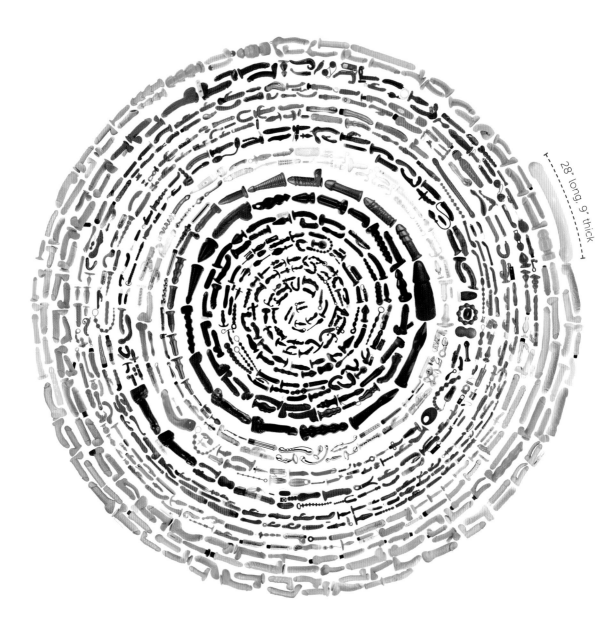

28" long, 9" thick

To read the sex toy sales analysis that accompanies these images, visit JonMillward.com/blog/rabbit.

22% Lube & Essentials

3% Gifts

3% Restraints

3% Dildos

4% Jiggle Balls

6% Cock Rings

5% Male Sex Toys

7% Anal Sex Toys

12% Lingerie

18% Vibrators

While
there are over
5,000 products of all
shapes, sizes and purposes,
83% of items sold belong to just
10 of the 40 main categories.

1. Lube & Essentials **2.** Vibrators
3. Lingerie **4.** Anal Sex Toys
5. Cock Rings **6.** Male Sex Toys
7. Jiggle Balls **8.** Dildos
9. Restraints
10. Gifts

47

VIBRATORS

HUM ARTIFICIALLY INTELLIGENT VIBRATOR BY DIMENSIONAL INDUSTRIES, INC.

2015

Medical-grade silicone

meethum.com

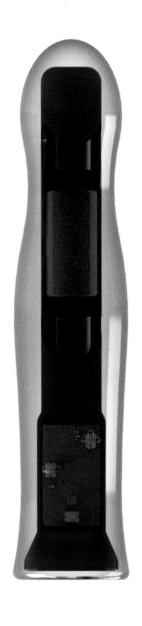

Those concerned about the threat of Artificial Intelligence (including smarty pants like Stephen Hawking and Bill Gates) take heed—the dawn of robotic sex is upon us. Over two years in development, the HUM vibrator is the brainchild of PhD physicists Jonathan Driscoll and Aaron Tynes Hammack and Sunny Allen, a cocktail waitress turned biohacker. Using technology that could run an atomic force microscope, HUM might sound a little overeducated, but what it can do is quite remarkable. This technology actually allows the vibrator to analyze the feedback response system of the human body. This precocious toy can sense your climax and respond in sync, drawing out and accentuating the experience.

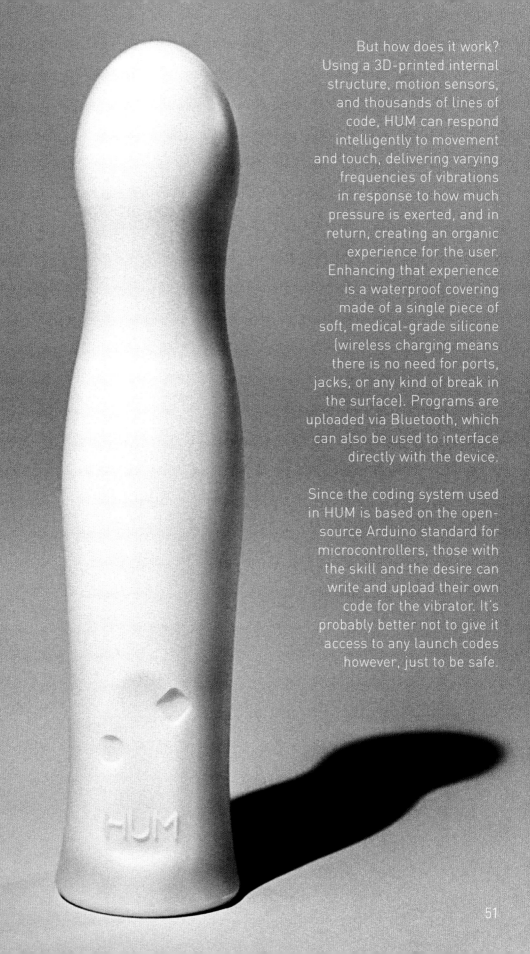

But how does it work? Using a 3D-printed internal structure, motion sensors, and thousands of lines of code, HUM can respond intelligently to movement and touch, delivering varying frequencies of vibrations in response to how much pressure is exerted, and in return, creating an organic experience for the user. Enhancing that experience is a waterproof covering made of a single piece of soft, medical-grade silicone (wireless charging means there is no need for ports, jacks, or any kind of break in the surface). Programs are uploaded via Bluetooth, which can also be used to interface directly with the device.

Since the coding system used in HUM is based on the open-source Arduino standard for microcontrollers, those with the skill and the desire can write and upload their own code for the vibrator. It's probably better not to give it access to any launch codes however, just to be safe.

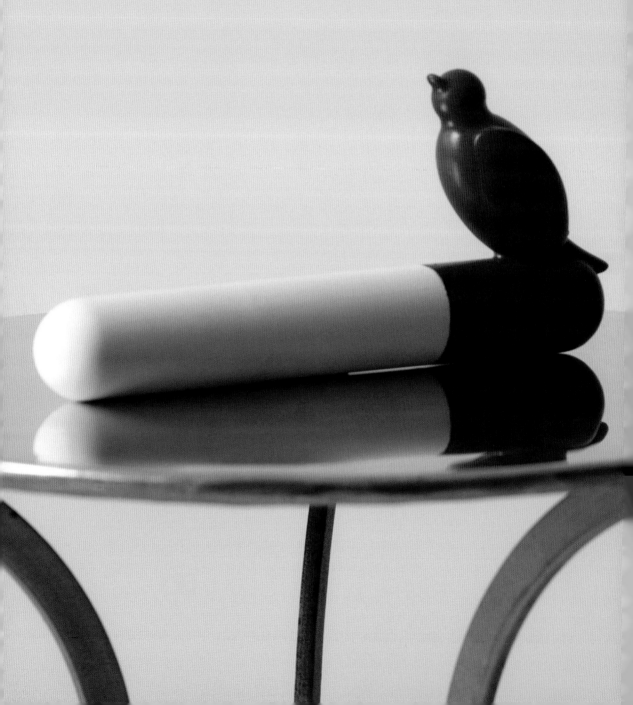

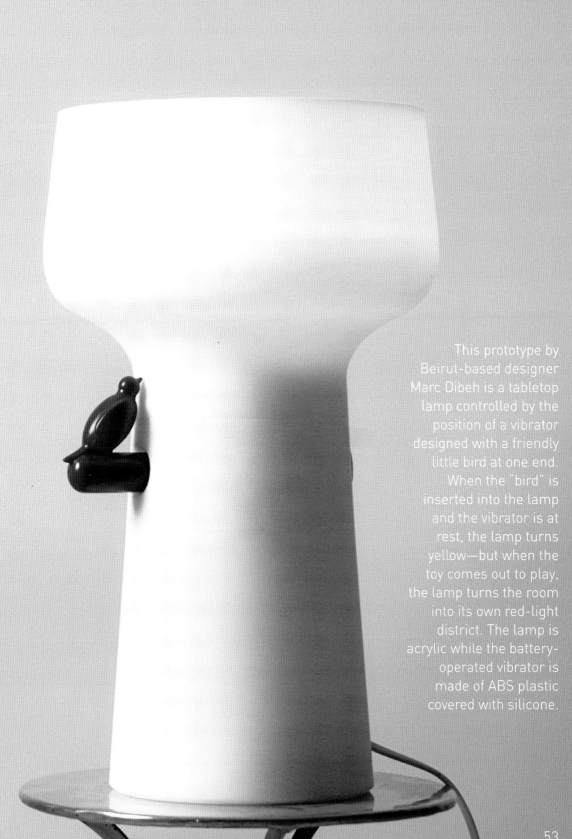

This prototype by Beirut-based designer Marc Dibeh is a tabletop lamp controlled by the position of a vibrator designed with a friendly little bird at one end. When the "bird" is inserted into the lamp and the vibrator is at rest, the lamp turns yellow—but when the toy comes out to play, the lamp turns the room into its own red-light district. The lamp is acrylic while the battery-operated vibrator is made of ABS plastic covered with silicone.

53

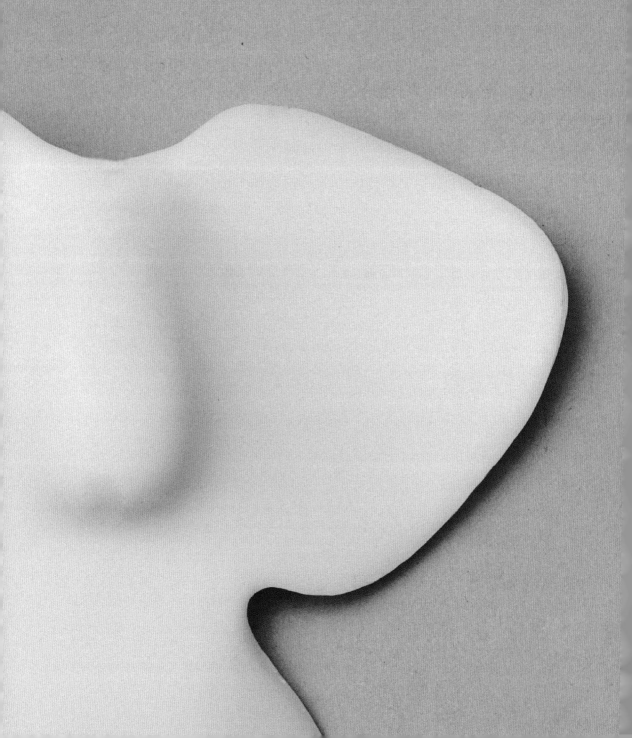

SONO LOVE
BY PATRYCJA DOMANSKA
2009
Silicone
patrycjadomanska.com

Inspired by the shape of both the fluid manta ray and the feminine orchid, the Sono Love vibrator is a prototype by Polish-born, Vienna-based designer Patrycja Domanska. The centralized cartridge of the soft silicone toy spreads the vibration across the entire surface, allowing it to become an extension of the hand. Sono Love deliberately comes with no instructions so the users can experience it in whichever way works best for them, alone or with company.

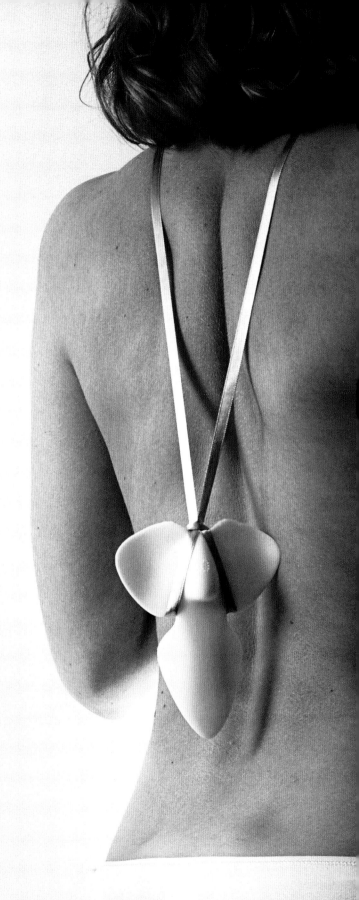

MOD OPEN-SOURCE VIBRATOR BY COMINGLE LLC

2014
Body-safe silicone
comingle.io

Founded in 2013 in Atlanta, Comingle designs and sells sex toys and DIY materials that encourage people to explore the intersection of sex and technology. After previously experimenting with a digital condom prototype, Comingle launched Mod, a multi-vibrating, open-source dildo. Mod is completely customizable by downloading apps from the company's website or by connecting plug-and-play controllers that sync it with your partner's heartbeat, connect it to your smartphone, or even change intensity based on movement in a video call.

Mod features three powerful, independently vibrating motors in a firm, flexible shaft made from 100 percent body-safe silicone. The multiple motors let Mod produce deep, rumbly vibrations (usually found in larger vibes) as well as simulate movement and other sensations.

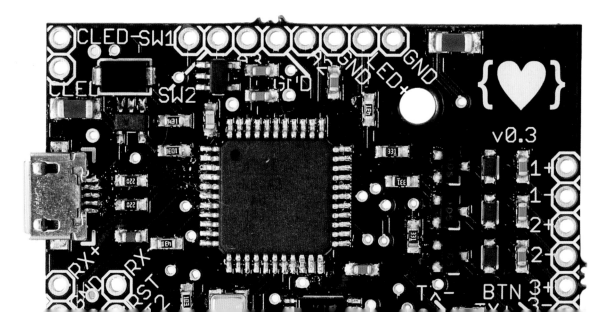

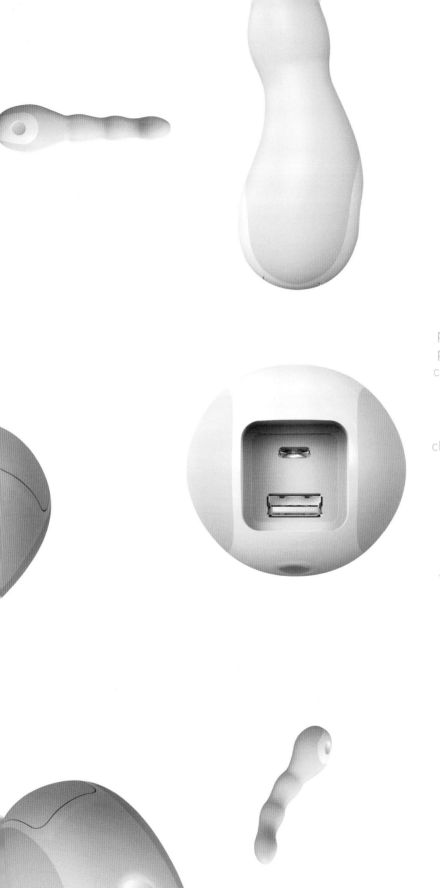
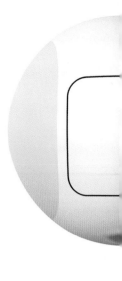

Since it's open-source, Mod's USB charging port can also be used for programming: users can create their own vibration patterns to share with others and change how Mod responds to button clicks, sensors, and other controllers. For the less tech-savvy, Mod also comes preprogrammed with its own patterns, or users can run new ones from the Comingle website. Real DIYers can take it a step further—Comingle provides all of the details to design your own Mod from scratch on their site.

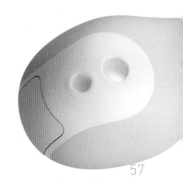

Q&A
ERIC KALÉN
FOUNDER AND
DESIGN DIRECTOR, TICKLER

What was your motivation for founding LELO?
I saw a great business opportunity and a great challenge to prove the power of design. LELO was my first contact with the sex toy business. The first toy I designed was the LELO Lily product.

How do people typically react when you tell them you design sex toys?
Most people are curious and positive about my job and what I do.

You said that "Tickler is for sex toys what H&M is for clothes." How do you keep the quality high with lower prices?
We keep the quality by making basic products and focusing on the key components like the materials and motors.

Are there certain toys that are more appealing to an older consumer vs. younger?
No, not necessarily, but it seems like consumers tend to spend more money on expensive toys when they know what they like.

You also design jewelry. Are any of your pieces designed to be used during sex?
Yes, I do but that´s more of a hobby.

What would you like to design next?
I collect Swedish crystal and one of my dream projects would be to design a collection for one of the famous Swedish glass manufacturers. Sweden has a long history of designing and manufacturing some of the finest crystal. I would love to be a part of that history and design functional glass, like consumer goods.

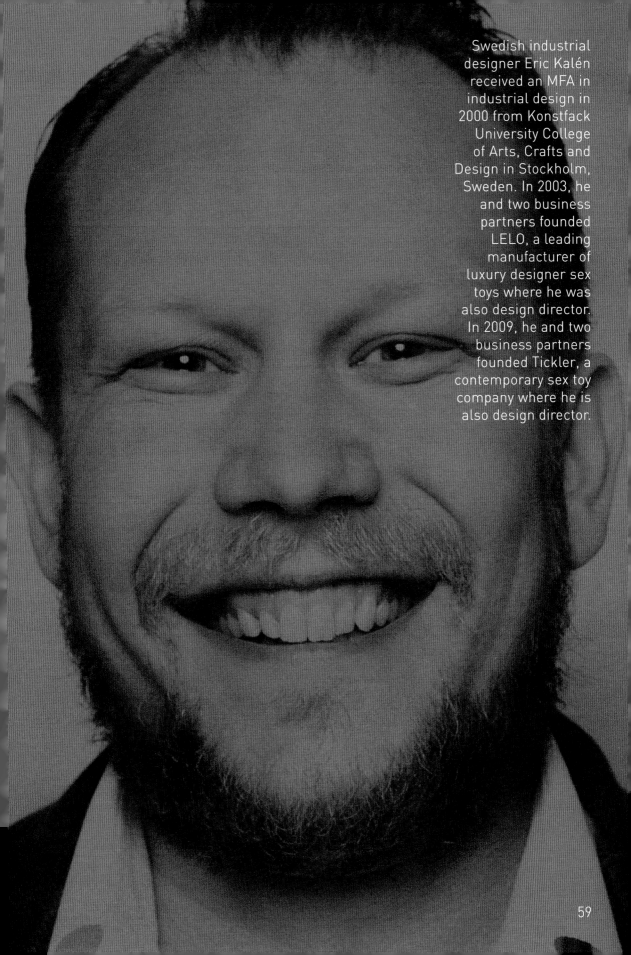

Swedish industrial designer Eric Kalén received an MFA in industrial design in 2000 from Konstfack University College of Arts, Crafts and Design in Stockholm, Sweden. In 2003, he and two business partners founded LELO, a leading manufacturer of luxury designer sex toys where he was also design director. In 2009, he and two business partners founded Tickler, a contemporary sex toy company where he is also design director.

POCKET & POWER TOYFRIENDS BY TICKLER

2013 (Pocket), 2010 (Power)
Body-safe silicone, ABS plastic
ticklervibes.com

These two collections from the Swedish brand Tickler prove that when it comes to vibrators, bigger isn't always better. Pocket Toyfriends are a set of four waterproof, mini-sized vibes for clitoral stimulation that are small enough to take along in your pocket or evening bag. Their bigger relatives, the Power Toyfriends, combine interesting shapes—one resembles a satellite disk, another a long-eared rabbit—with a choice of speeds and pulsations to create their own unique sensations. Both collections come in a choice of red, black, yellow, or blue, depending on the form that appeals most to the user.

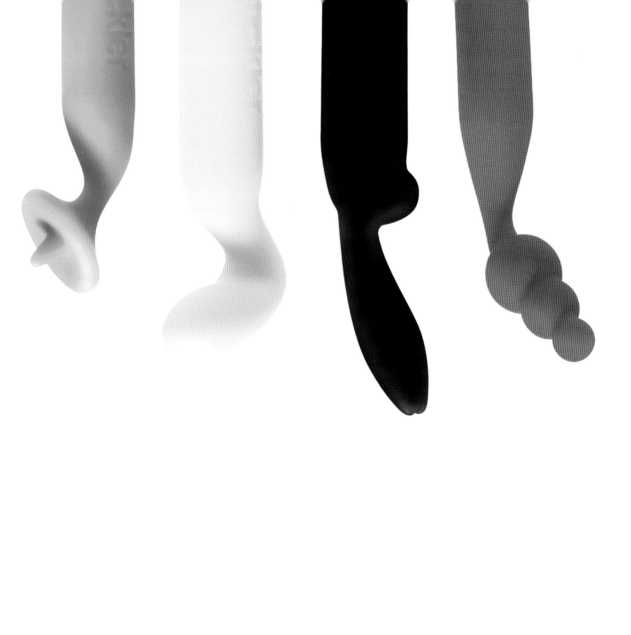
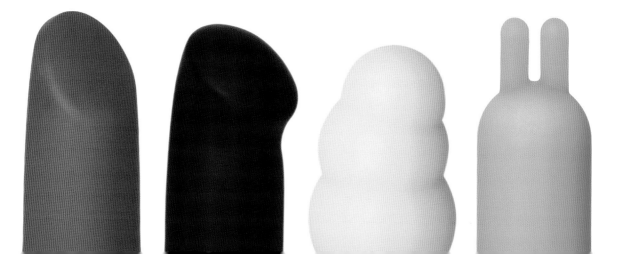

IROHA
MIDORI, SAKURA & YUKI
BY TENGA

2013
FDA-approved, food-grade silicone
iroha-tenga.com

According to the Japanese
sex toy makers at Tenga (best
known for their egg-shaped
male strokers), the iroha
brand is "created by women
for women." Included in the
collection are three friendly
sisters named Yuki, Midori,
and Sakura. Each palm-size,
fleshy orb works both as a
vibrator and erogenous
zone massager.

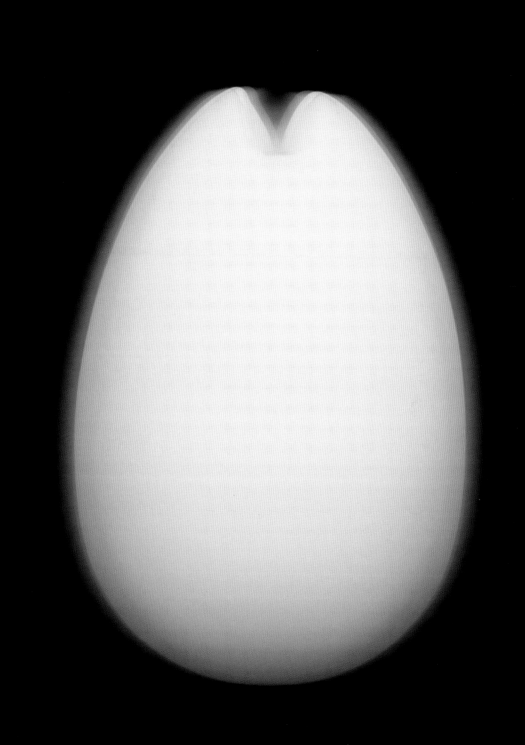

Snowman-shaped Yuki is
semi-insertable, while the
other two are intended for
clitoral stimulation. Midori
has a softly rounded nob
on top to help better
pinpoint your pleasure,
while Sukura has an
adjustable, indented
tip at the end for more
intense sensation.

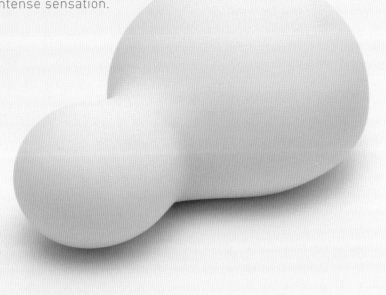
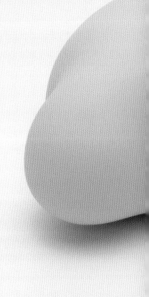

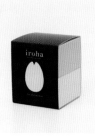
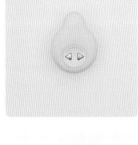
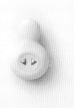
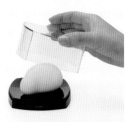
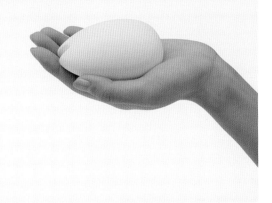

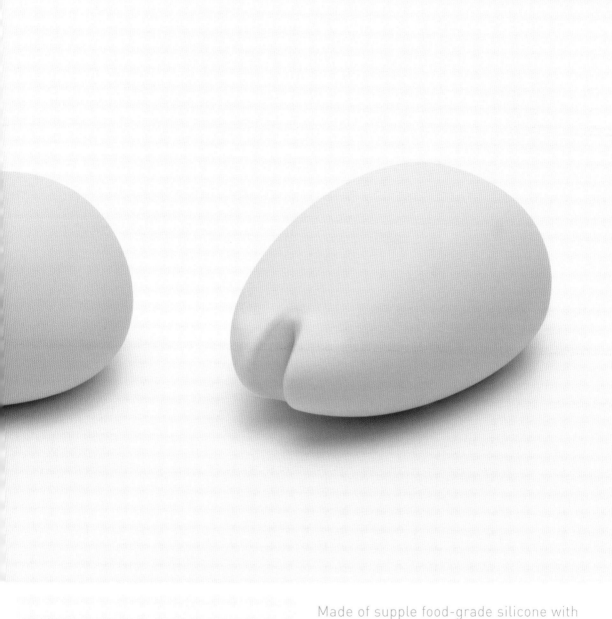

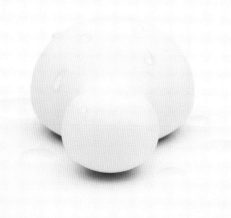

Made of supple food-grade silicone with an anti-dust coating to help keep them clean, the rechargeable, water-resistant vibrators have a two-button control and work on a magnetic charging base. To borrow the Japanese word for cute, these are some seriously *kawaii* vibes.

SMILE MAKERS
BY RAMBLIN' BRANDS LTD.

2012

FDA-approved, body-safe silicone

smilemakerscollection.com

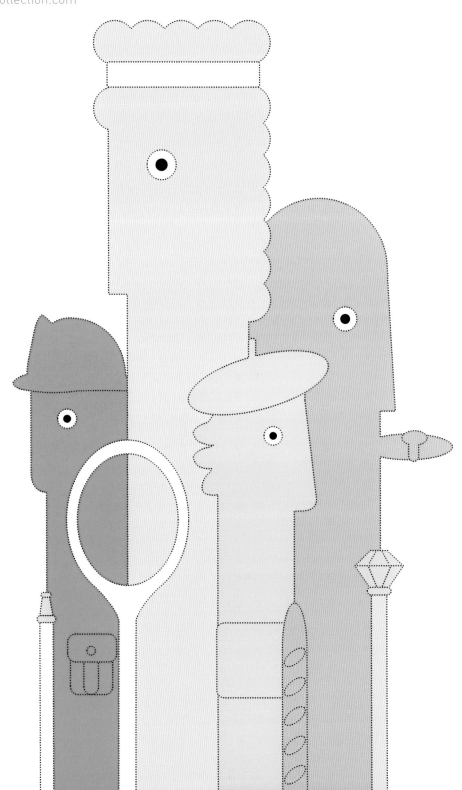

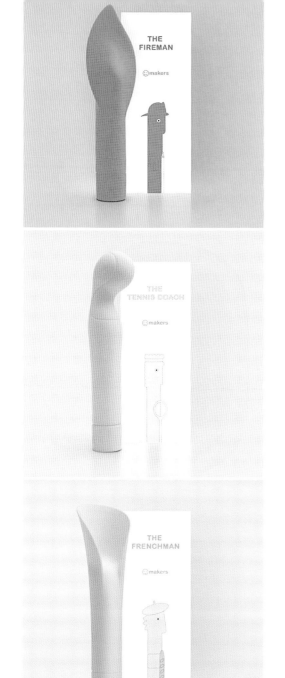

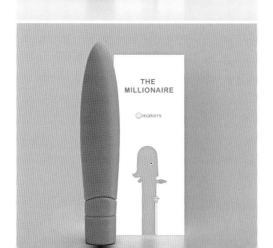

Smile Makers is a family of battery-operated vibrators intended to be sold not as sex toys but as beauty care products, in the same way skin care, cosmetics, or fragrance products are sold. To make the products more approachable for those who might not have purchased a vibrator previously, Ramblin' Brands hired creative partner Micah Walker, who thought injecting some humor into the design would help relieve any anxiety about the purchase. As a result, four stereotypical "female fantasies" were selected for the vibrators that would work across as many cultures as possible.

The team partnered with Ian Swanson and Achille Lenglemetz, who came up with the actual vibrator shapes based on the four fantasy concepts. The Fireman is a flame-shaped clitoral stimulator, The Millionaire is a cigar-shaped vibrator, The Frenchman has a flared tip to simulate oral sex, and The Tennis Coach is a gentle G-spot vibrator with a ball-shaped knob at the end. The humor extends to the packaging design as well, which includes illustrations of the characters that inspired each of the forms.

REVEL BODY SOL
BY REVEL BODY

2014
High-grade polycarbonate, body-safe
silicone, gold-plated contacts
revelbody.com

Since an orgasm is also known as
la petite mort, or "the little death,"
then fans of *Star Wars* might call the
Revel Body SOL the "little Death Star."
Unlike other battery-operated devices
that use rotary vibration motors, the
core of the orb-shaped SOL uses a
linear motor that provides pulsation
along the length of the product.
Intended for body massage or clitoral
stimulation, SOL claims to be the
only vibrator that operates at 136.1
Hz (a.k.a., the "frequency of Om"), a
sacred frequency recognized by many
ancient cultures as the energy that
connects and joins all things together.

You don't have to be a yogi master to
enjoy SOL however—you can simply
use the Om pre-setting. Completely
waterproof, SOL is also designed
to provide underwater suction and
vibration when using the "backside" of
the device. SOL is also travel-friendly
with a USB-rechargeable lithium
ion polymer battery, and comes with
several removable attachments for
different sensations.

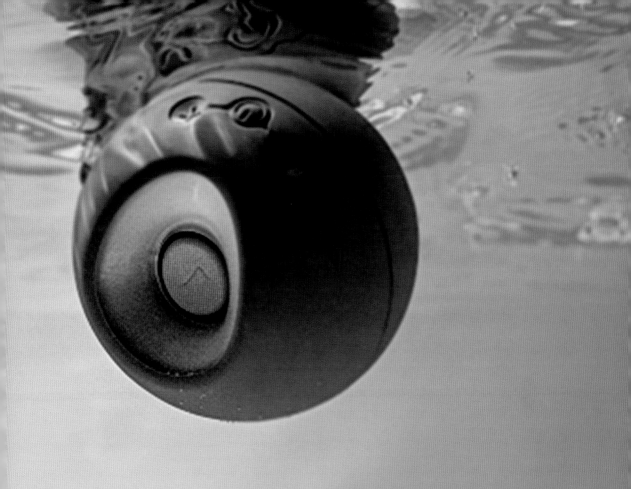

LOVELIFE COLLECTION BY OHMIBOD

2013
Body-safe silicone, polyurethane-
coated ABS plastic
ohmibod.com

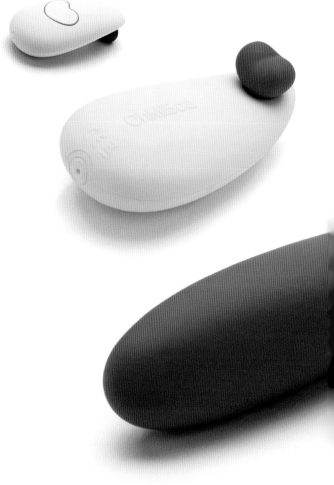

The Red Dot Design Award–winning
Lovelife collection, which includes kegel
weights (page 36) and the Share couples
ring (page 158), is OhMiBod's first line
of standard vibrators. Resembling a
half-peeled banana, the Adventure
Triple Stim vibe (far right) offers three
powerful motors for clitoral, internal,
and anal stimulation. Using the heart-
shaped control panel (with buttons that
look like two eyes and a mouth) you can
cycle through the line's preset scalable
pulsation patterns.

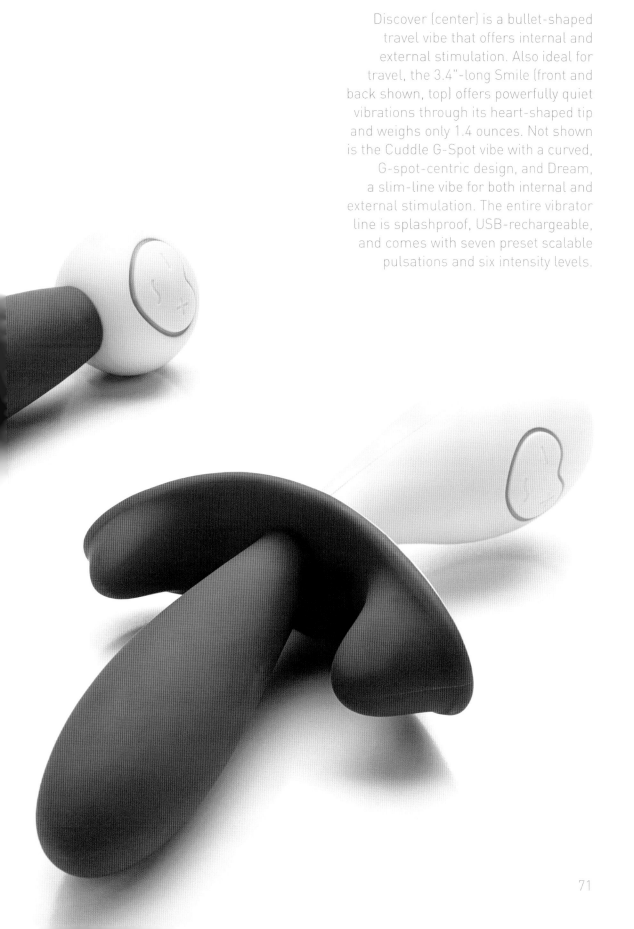

Discover (center) is a bullet-shaped travel vibe that offers internal and external stimulation. Also ideal for travel, the 3.4"-long Smile (front and back shown, top) offers powerfully quiet vibrations through its heart-shaped tip and weighs only 1.4 ounces. Not shown is the Cuddle G-Spot vibe with a curved, G-spot-centric design, and Dream, a slim-line vibe for both internal and external stimulation. The entire vibrator line is splashproof, USB-rechargeable, and comes with seven preset scalable pulsations and six intensity levels.

71

LIMON
BY MINNA LIFE

2013
Medical-grade silicone,
stainless-steel charging pins
minnalife.com

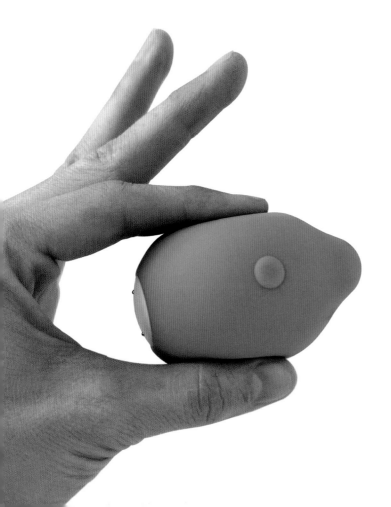

Squeezing lemons might help
make lemonade, but squeezing
a Limon can make something
even sweeter. Using Minna
Life's revolutionary squeeze
technology (simply put, the harder
you squeeze, the stronger the
vibrations) Limon offers the ability
to compose, record, and play back
custom vibration patterns for
clitoral or body massage.

Designed particularly for couples
use but also good for singles,
Limon is the first platform
for Minna's Rumble Motor
Technology, which concentrates
vibrations in the tip to create
rumbly (rather than numbing and
buzzy) vibrations. Weighing only
2.7 ounces and measuring 3" x
2" x 2", Limon is waterproof (but
not dishwasher-safe) and comes
in the noncitrusy colors of pink
or teal. Limon's handy, USB-
compatible magnetic charging
dock can also be used as a stand,
so you can always have your own
sexy farmers' market right on
your bedside table.

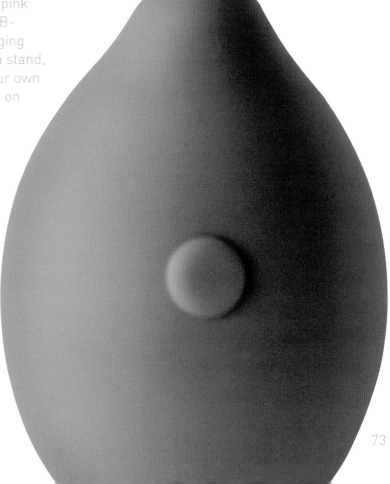

TARA
BY LELO

2013
Body-safe silicone, ABS plastic
lelo.com

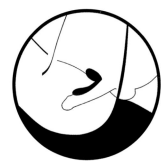

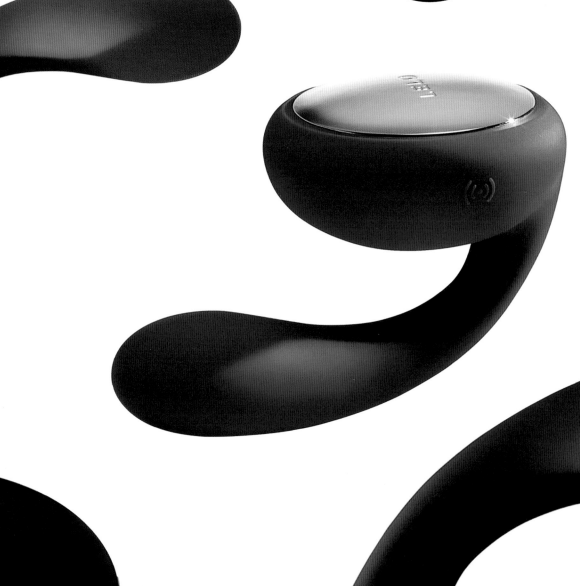

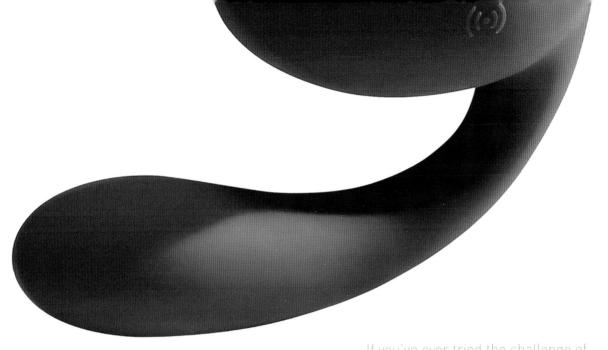

If you've ever tried the challenge of rubbing your stomach while patting your head, you have the gist of how the TARA vibe works. Worn inside the vagina during intercourse, TARA is a waterproof, USB-rechargeable couples massager that combines vibrations and rotations for both partners. The phallic end of the toy is inserted into the vagina for a G-spot massage, and a penis or dildo is then inserted underneath the toy as it rotates, pressing it up against the G-spot during intercourse. At the same time, an external, disk-shaped stimulator vibrates above the clitoris and can be felt by both partners. A one-button interface controls six vibration/rotation modes for the device. A similar product from LELO, called IDA, offers comparable functionality along with a remote control feature.

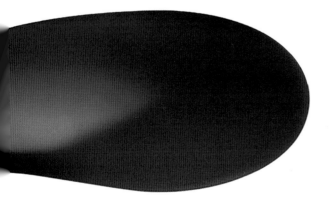

SMART WAND BY LELO

2012
Body-safe silicone, ABS plastic
lelo.com

Available in a medium or large version, the Red Dot Design Award–winning SMART WAND vibrator resembles the wand-style body massagers found on display at mainstream retailers like Brookstone. Claimed to be the most powerful cordless wand massager on the market, the 12"-long SMART WAND Large offers a deeply resonant vibe in eight vibration patterns in adjustable speeds. At 8.7", the SMART WAND Medium is better suited for travel and offers two hours of use from a full charge. Both use LELO's SenseTouch technology, a tactile response function that increases vibrations on skin contact.

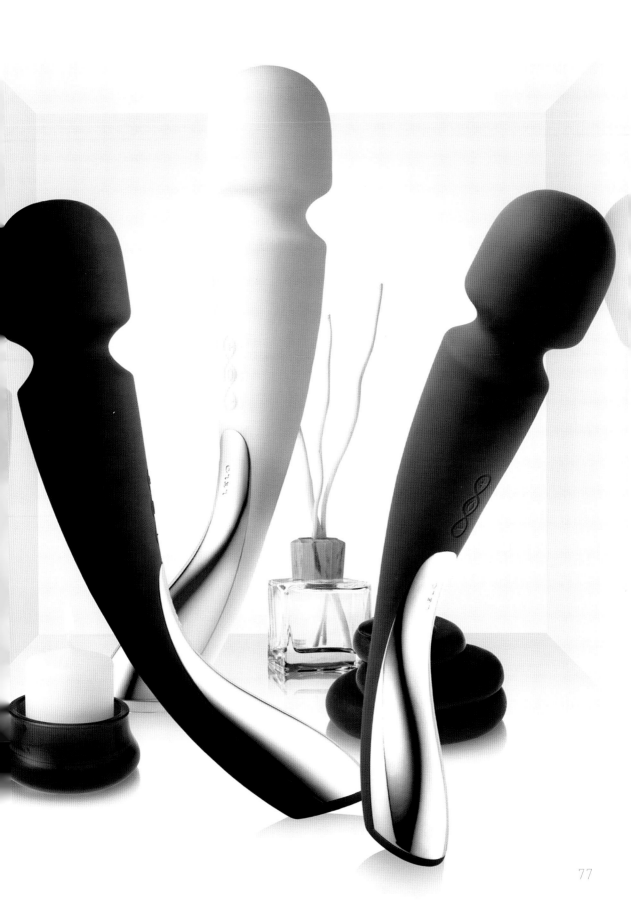

Q&A
MOLLY MURPHY
DIRECTOR OF SALES & MARKETING, JIMMYJANE

Your founder Ethan Imboden left day-to-day operations at Jimmyjane in February 2014 after it was acquired by pleasure-product-centric holdings company Diamond Products. Can you tell us a bit how Imboden began Jimmyjane's award-winning collaboration with Yves Béhar?
Ethan Imboden founded the company in 2003, seeing an unprecedented opportunity to transform consumer experience in an area of universal interest—sexuality. Ethan took many by surprise (including himself) when he announced that he would be launching a brand focused on pleasure.

Ethan and Yves have known each other for years from San Francisco and the world of design. FORM 2 was the first launch of Pleasure to the People, a groundbreaking series of waterproof, rechargeable vibrators designed by the friends and creative conspirators, which was then followed by FORM 3 and FORM 4.

When the collaboration commenced in 2007, the brief called for the development of a single product. However, as work got underway, the two designers discovered there were numerous opportunities they wanted to explore. The project was expanded to a series of three distinctive designs and innovations, each with a unique power to please.

Are you currently working with any other outside designers? What are the benefits/challenges to working with an outside firm?
After the Pleasure to the People series Jimmyjane launched the Hello Touch wearable vibrator, designed in-house. At the heart of Jimmyjane is a design studio, and currently the company is leveraging their veteran team of designers for the next round of products in the design cycle. As a design-centric brand the company enjoys partnering with various creatives on collaborations. Partnerships with Yves Béhar, W Hotels Worldwide, and artist Jamie Hewlett of Gorillaz disrupt the category, open up the brand to new audiences, and change the public's perception of pleasure products. One of the challenges of collaborations is the combination of two creative teams. While it forces both teams to see the subject in a new light, it can sometimes slow the process. With Yves Béhar we were lucky enough to have both teams in San Francisco, which made communication and collaboration easy, but that isn't always the case and sometimes the distance between two teams stalls the design process.

Since you launched in 2004, what has been the single-most important improvement to the sex toy industry?
The shift in the public's perception of vibrators is the most important change we have seen. Once stigmatized, consumers now recognize vibrators for the positive effects a quality product can have on their sex lives and relationships.

How do you test your products?
We conduct rigorous testing in-house to ensure our products meet quality standards. All of our products are made with 100 percent body-safe, nontoxic materials. We enlist third party testing and certification in the US (FCC, ETL, and UL) and also adhere to strict EU regulations (CE and RoHS). All Jimmyjane designs are created with an emphasis on quality and long product lifecycle, which we back with an unparalleled three-year warranty.

Which is your most popular line of products?
Our line of FORM waterproof rechargeable vibrators is our flagship line. Our Hello Touch wearable vibrator, launched in 2013, is part of a new line and has also quickly become a top seller.

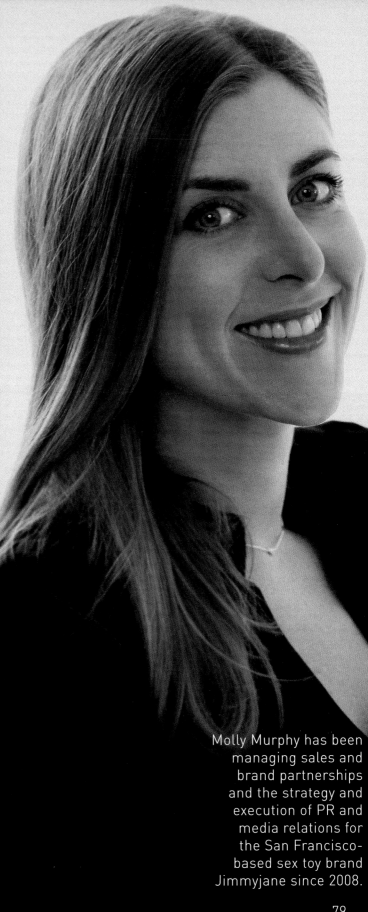

What kind of demographics about your customers could you share with us?
Our products appeal to a mass audience and we see consumers across all demographics. Currently if you look at our website we have a split of 55 percent males/45 percent female consumers. We are seeing the most interest from between the ages of twenty-five and thirty-four, however our biggest purchasers are women forty-five to sixty-five-plus.

The Hello Touch has been well received. What inspired this very different approach to vibration?
We knew that the couples market was growing and research showed foreplay is a very important part of connection and the sexual experience. With Hello Touch we wanted to create something that was very intuitive to use and would enhance how you would normally touch a partner. Hello Touch is an extension to the experience couples are already having and enhances how they connect and engage in foreplay. Our engineers worked hard to ensure the Vibration Pods were powerful, yet had a thin profile, so you can move uninhibited. Because of the mobility of the fingers you can touch, massage, and pleasure erogenous zones unlike with other vibrators. Additionally, both partners are very much a part of the experience; it is still your partner's touch and movement delivering pleasure, which sustains the connection element.

Molly Murphy has been managing sales and brand partnerships and the strategy and execution of PR and media relations for the San Francisco-based sex toy brand Jimmyjane since 2008.

FORM
BY JIMMYJANE

2007 (FORM 6), 2009 (FORM 2), 2010
(FORM 3), 2011 (FORM 4, shown here), 2015 (FORM 5)
Medical-grade silicone
jimmyjane.com

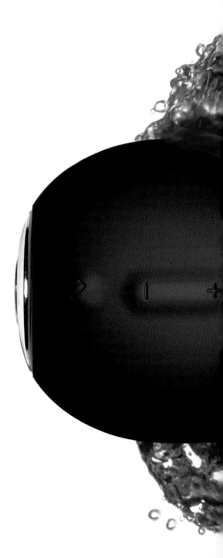

The FORM series of rechargeable vibrators was
first launched in 2010 as the Pleasure to the People
collection by Jimmyjane founder Ethan Imboden
and industrial designer Yves Béhar of the San
Francisco-based design firm Fuseproject. This trio
of waterproof, body-hugging vibes includes the
IDEA Award-winning, dual-motor FORM 2 (a dead
ringer for the USS Enterprise), the tongue-shaped
FORM 3, and the more traditionally shaped FORM
4, nicknamed the "Barry White" of vibrators by
Jimmyjane for its deep, rumbling vibration.

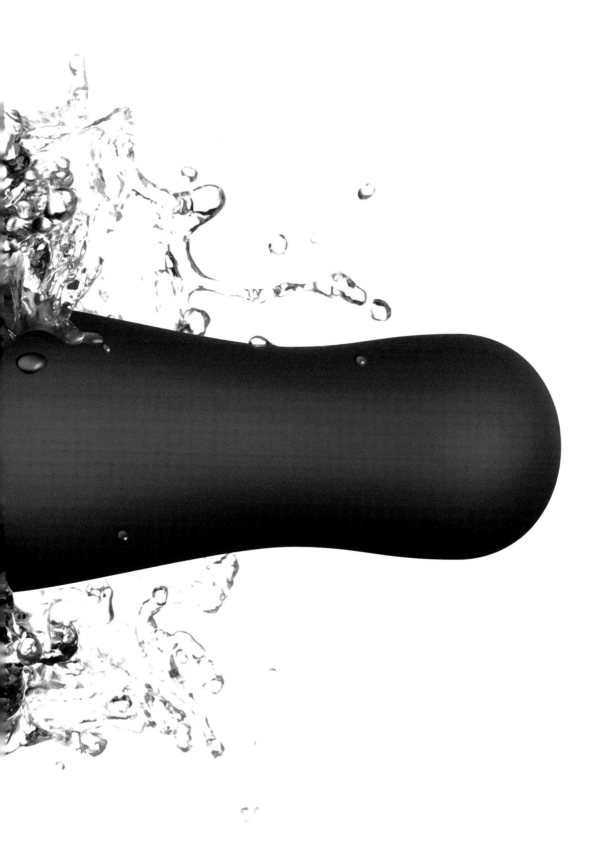

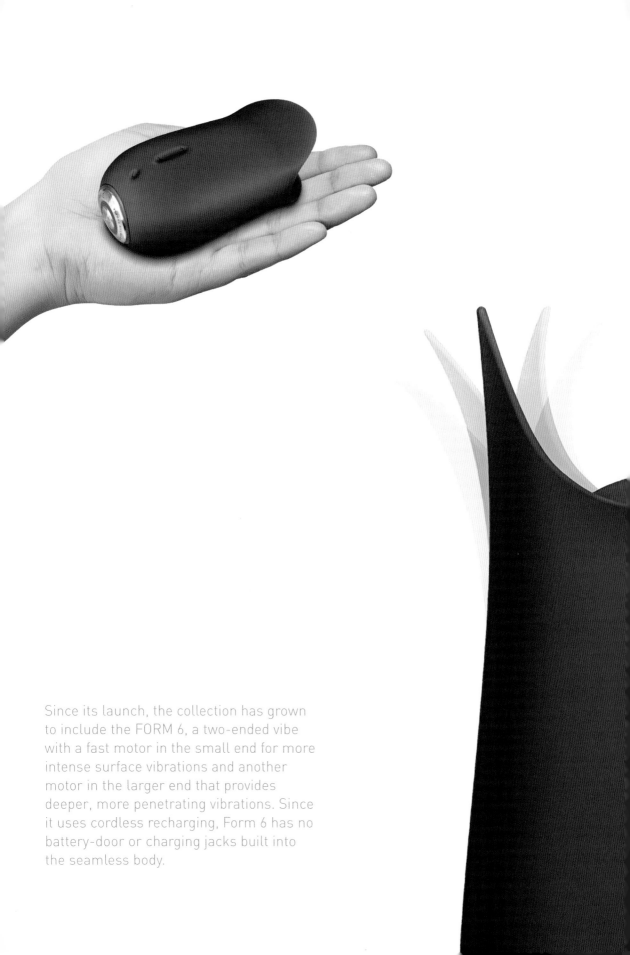

Since its launch, the collection has grown
to include the FORM 6, a two-ended vibe
with a fast motor in the small end for more
intense surface vibrations and another
motor in the larger end that provides
deeper, more penetrating vibrations. Since
it uses cordless recharging, Form 6 has no
battery-door or charging jacks built into
the seamless body.

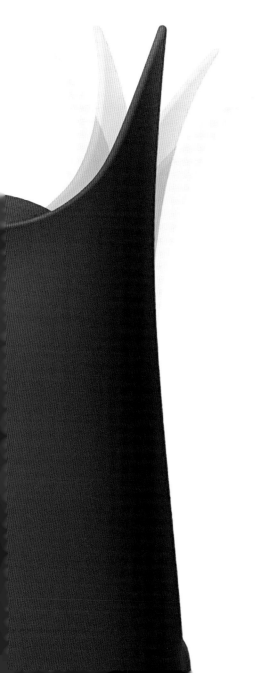

The latest introduction, FORM 5 (the product numbers are not in consecutive order), is claimed to be the first vibrator optimized to stimulate both the clitoris and the sensitive areas surrounding it known as the labia majora. Designed in-house by Jimmyjane's veteran team of designers—most notably VP of Creative Development Peter Caropelo—the USB-rechargeable FORM 5 (shown center and top left) features a cylindrical shape with a powerful motor that creates a direct, rumbling vibration. The motor lies beneath a bulbous tip named the "pleasure dome" surrounded by two supple silicone "pleasure wings" that can either stimulate the surrounding areas of the labia or be used directly on the clitoris to create a sensation similar to oral sex. It can also be placed on the base of the penis with the wings hugging the shaft.

DUET LUX
BY CRAVE

2013
Body-safe silicone, 24k gold plating
lovecrave.com

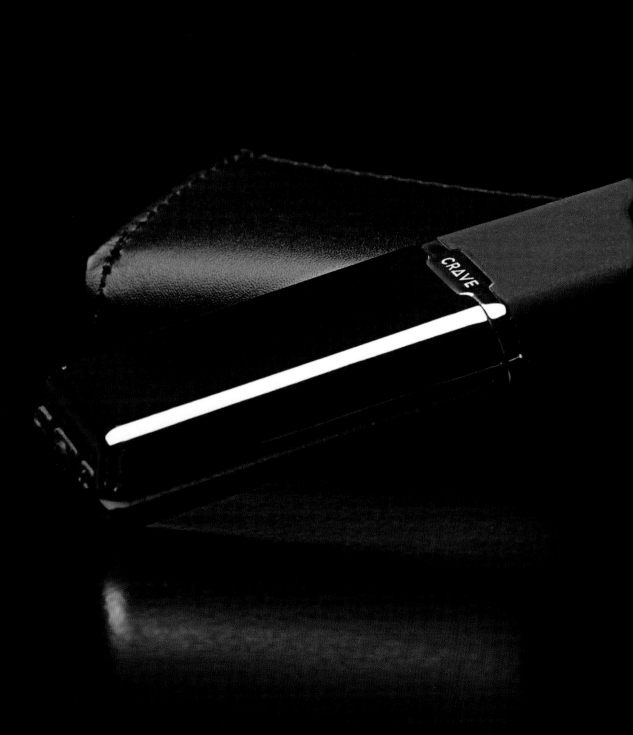

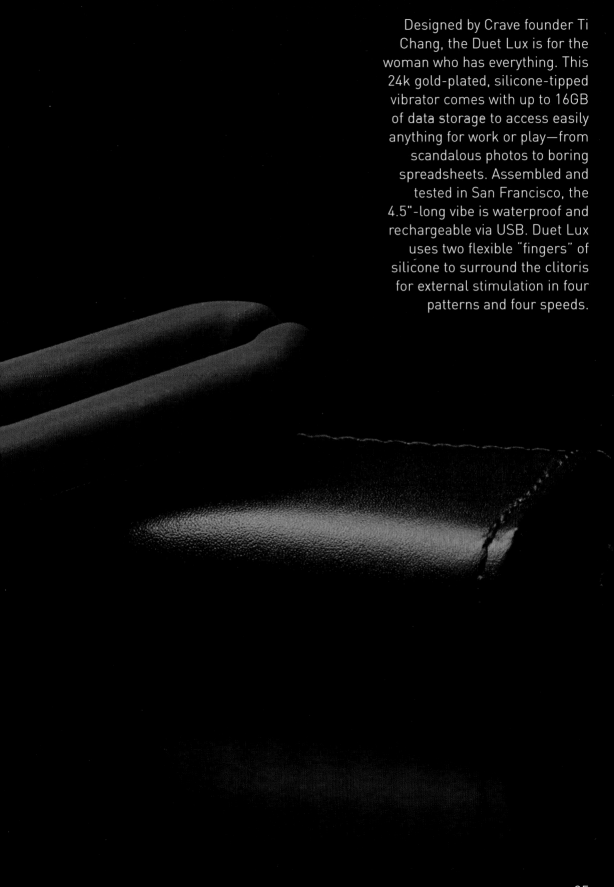

Designed by Crave founder Ti Chang, the Duet Lux is for the woman who has everything. This 24k gold-plated, silicone-tipped vibrator comes with up to 16GB of data storage to access easily anything for work or play—from scandalous photos to boring spreadsheets. Assembled and tested in San Francisco, the 4.5"-long vibe is waterproof and rechargeable via USB. Duet Lux uses two flexible "fingers" of silicone to surround the clitoris for external stimulation in four patterns and four speeds.

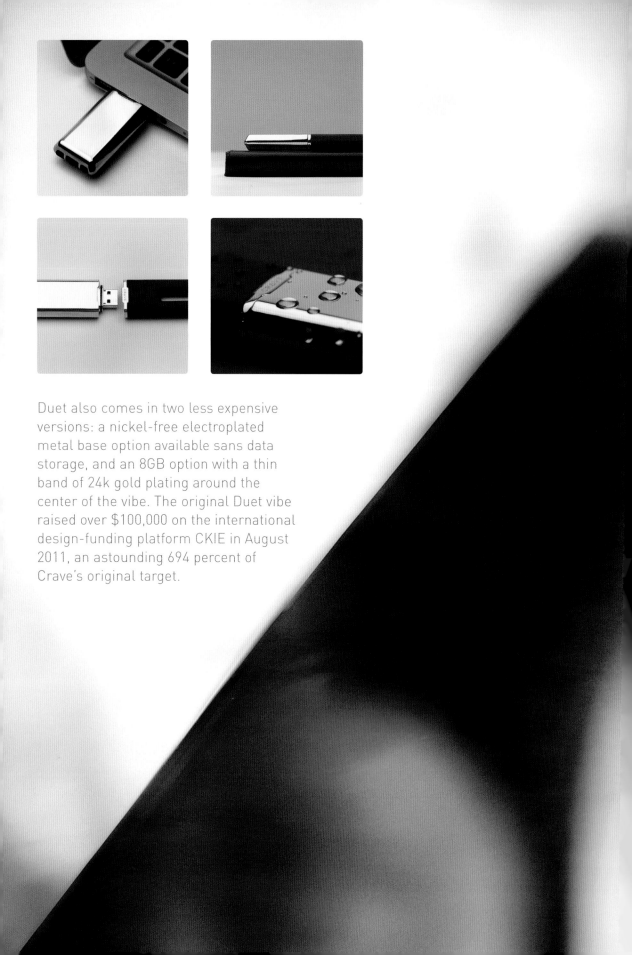

Duet also comes in two less expensive versions: a nickel-free electroplated metal base option available sans data storage, and an 8GB option with a thin band of 24k gold plating around the center of the vibe. The original Duet vibe raised over $100,000 on the international design-funding platform CKIE in August 2011, an astounding 694 percent of Crave's original target.

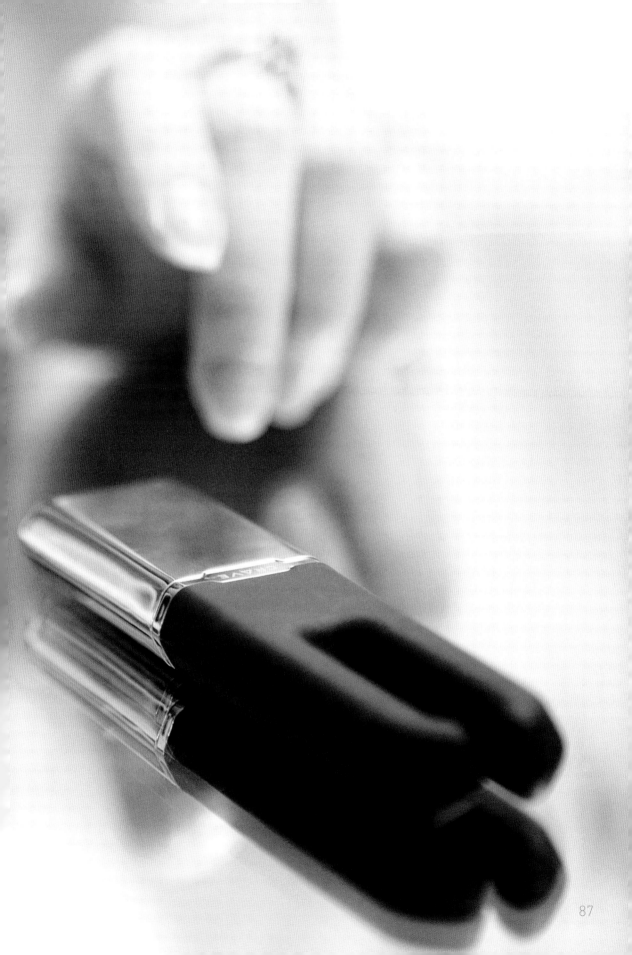

VI-BO
BY TENGA

2013
Thermoplastic elastomer, ABS plastic
tenga-global.com

Tenga's first line of couples vibrators, Vi-Bo is centered around a small vibrating orb that inserts into different thermoplastic elastomer cases for vaginal, clitoral, and erogenous zone massage. Vi-Bo's playful colors and shapes, easy push-button control, and medium speed make it ideal for couples just starting out with toys.

The waterproof collection includes a Finger Orb, Ring Orb (to be worn on the shaft of the penis), Hand Orb (worn across the palm to free up the fingers), dual-sided Twin Orb, and Stick Orb. Though the battery-operated orbs easily pop out of their cases for cleaning, users are warned *not* to insert them directly into the body like one would Ben Wa balls.

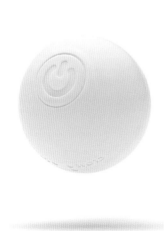

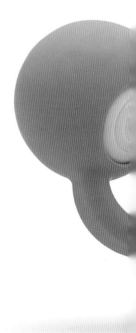

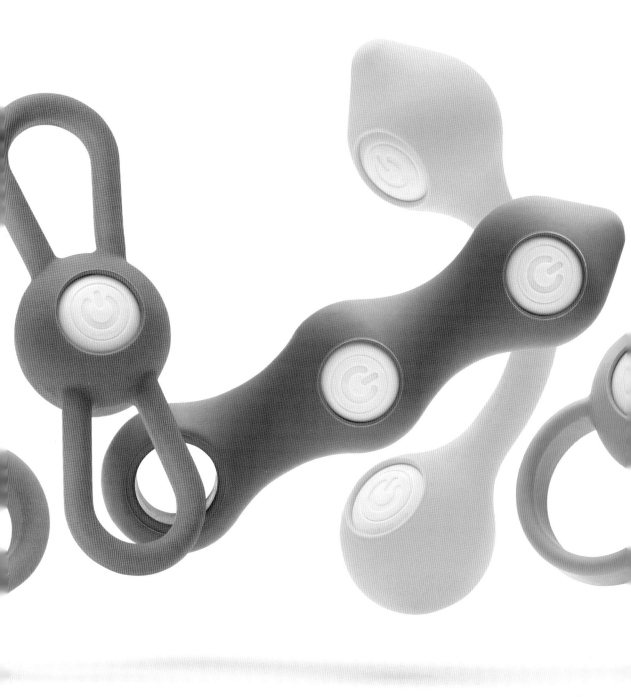

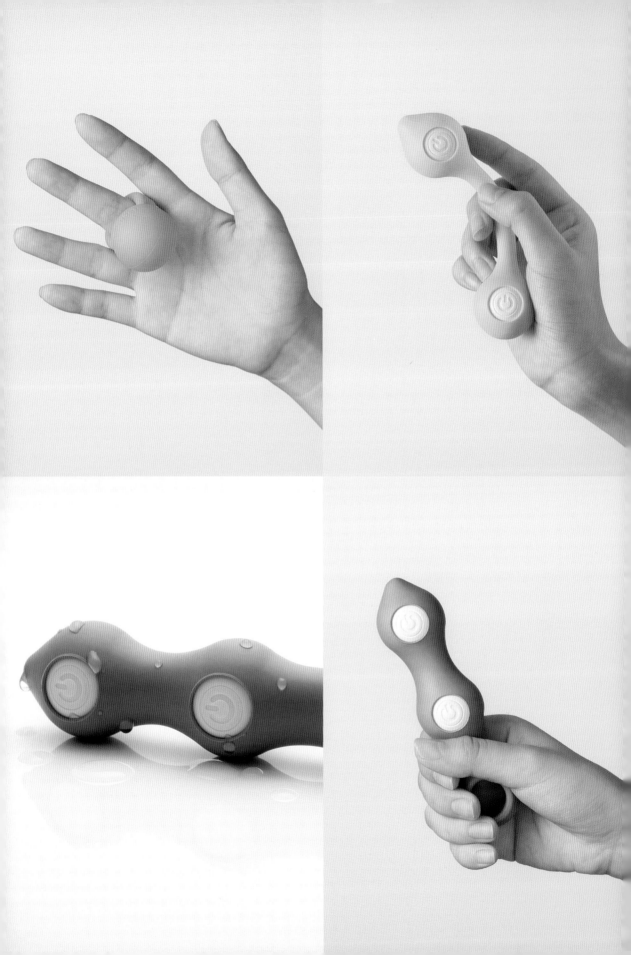

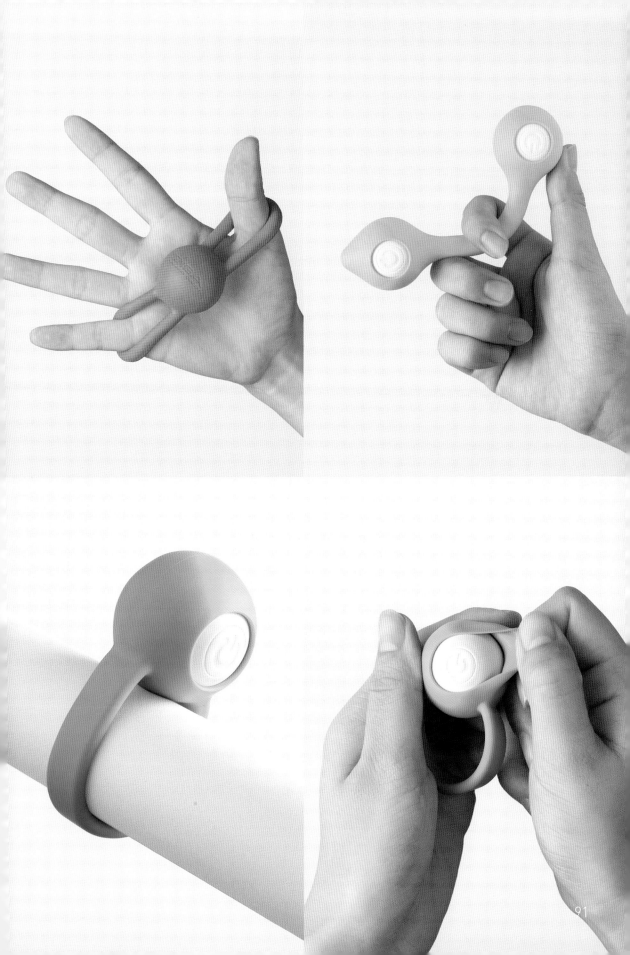

HELLO TOUCH
BY JIMMYJANE

2013 (Hello Touch), 2015 (Hello Touch X)
Body-safe silicone, stainless steel (Hello Touch X pods)
jimmyjane.com

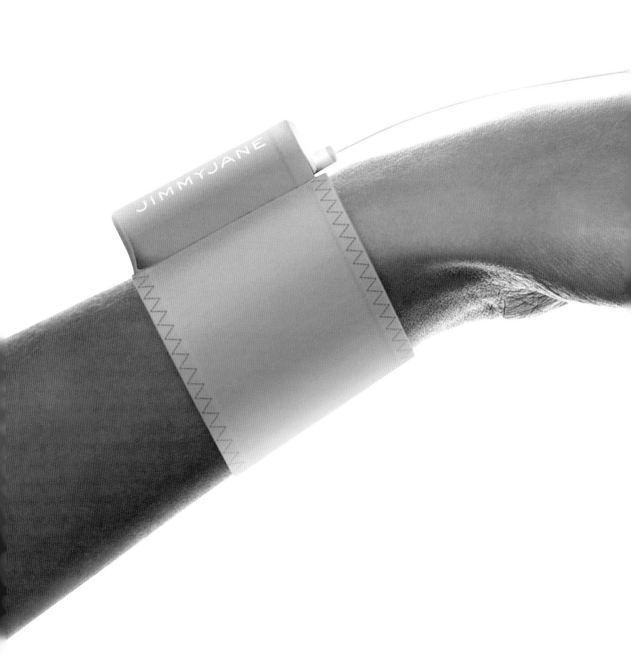

Jimmyjane entered a new category in 2013 with their cyber-sexy Hello Touch fingertip vibrators. Designed to deliver over three times the power in less than one third of the size of other fingertip vibrators, Hello Touch is also claimed to be the only device optimized for both internal and clitoral stimulation.

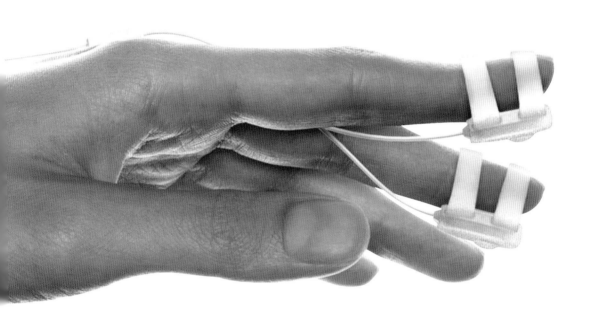

To administer a "friendly" touch, the user slips the power source on his or her wrist, pushes the On button, and wraps the two supple silicone fingerpad vibration pods on the fingers of choice. Shower-ready and washable, they can be used to stimulate the clitoris, G-spot, nipples, and any other spot reachable with the fingers. If having the vibrators on the front of your fingertips starts to make it difficult to feel what you are after, you can try placing them on the back of the fingertips, which then turns the fingers themselves into the vibration source.

In 2014 Jimmyjane launched Hello Touch X, the company's second generation of wearable vibrators intended to introduce electro stimulation play (also referred to as E-stim) to the masses. Hello Touch X comes with an improved power button set-up and two sets of pods, one for vibration and one for E-stim. When the two E-stim finger pods come in contact with the body, a light current of electrons passes between them to create sensations ranging from a light tingling to intense pulse waves, similar to those created by TENS and EMS machines used in physical therapy for pain management. For those unfamiliar with E-stim, it's extremely important to understand all of the risks involved, and users should do their due diligence beyond any one manufacturer's safety instructions.

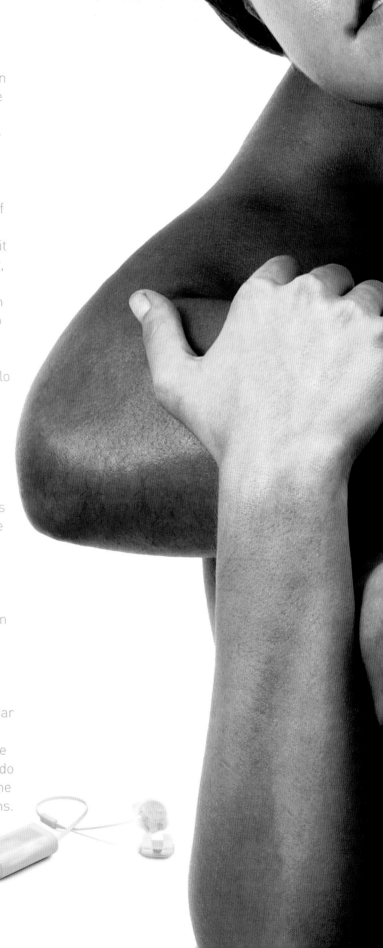

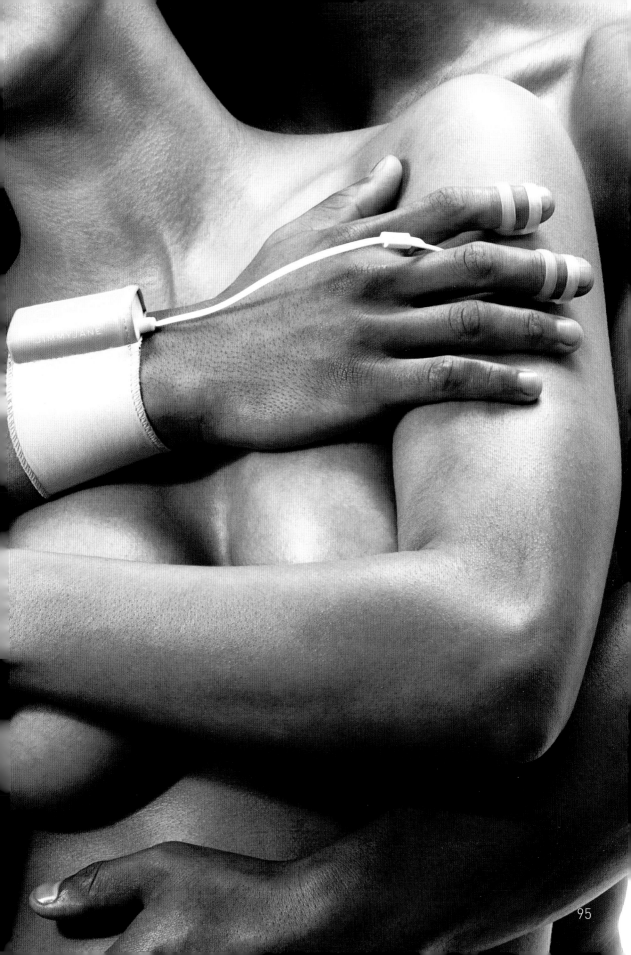

INA WAVE
BY LELO

2014
Body-safe silicone
lelo.com

The rabbit, known for its prolific breeding ability,
is also the name of one of the most iconic vibrator
shapes in the industry. With the INA WAVE (shown
on the opposite page in pink), LELO has taken the
basic rabbit shape (a long G-spot massager and an
short, external clitoral stimulator) and added a back
and forth "come hither" finger-like motion for the
internal arm.

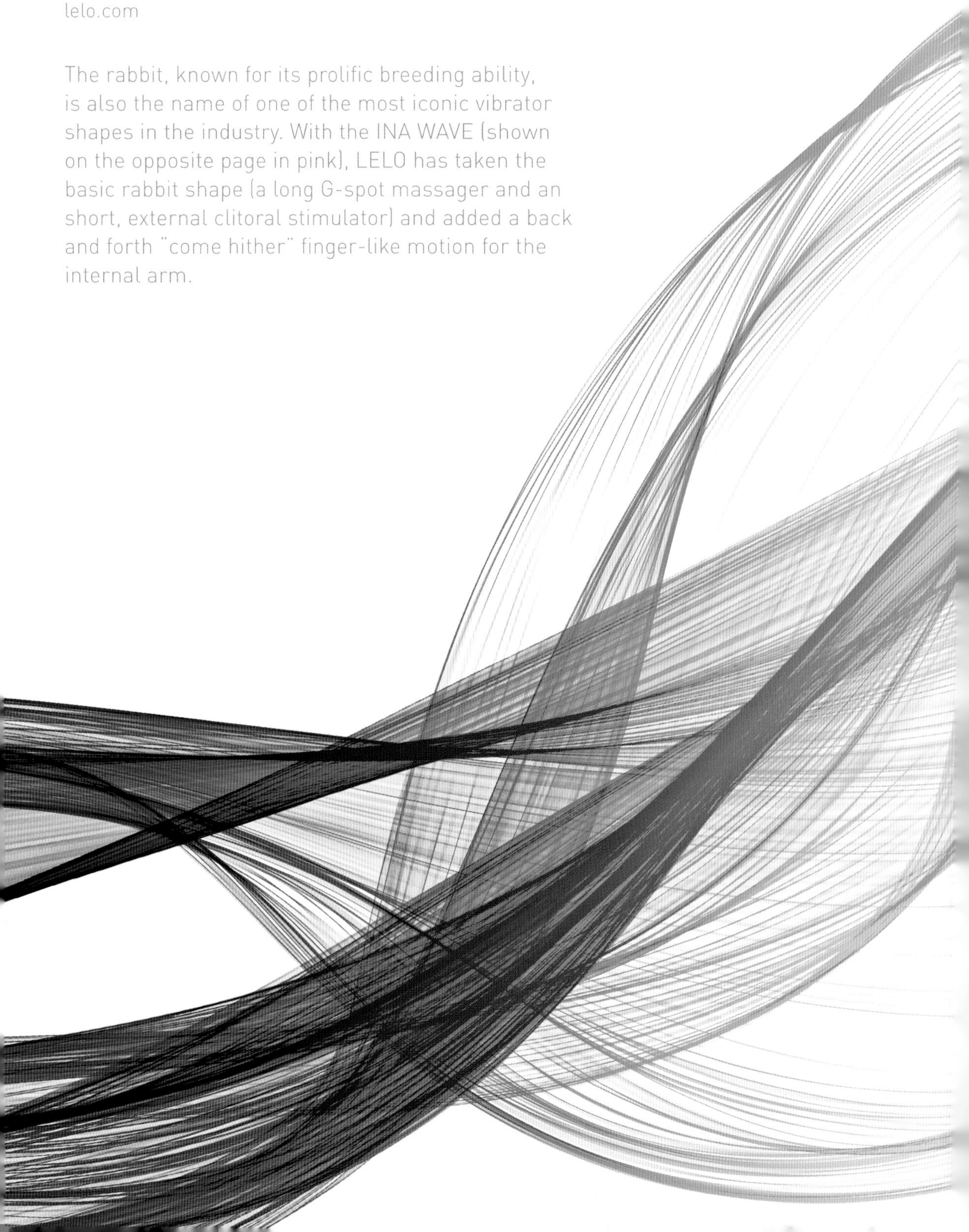

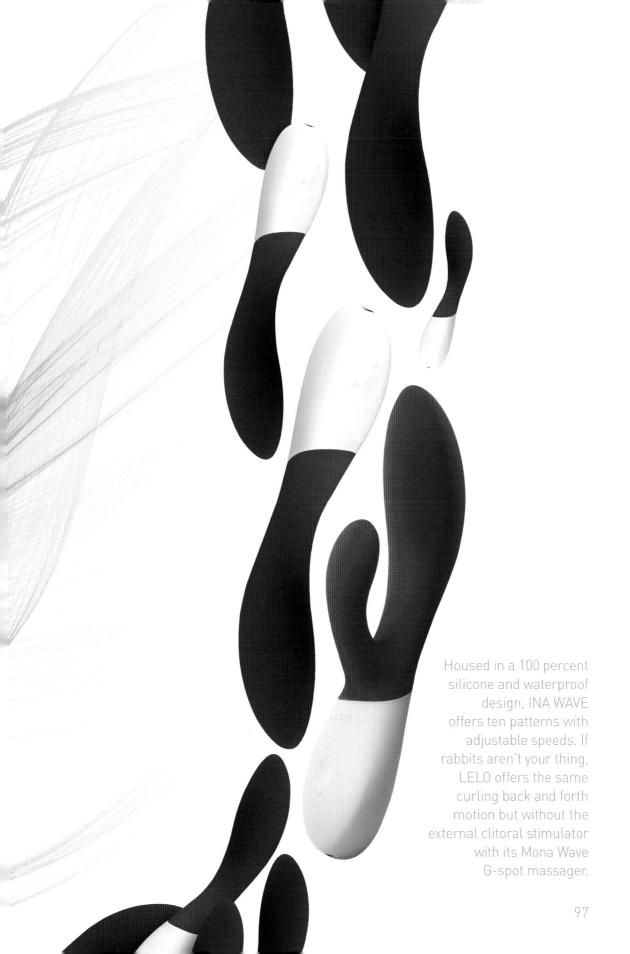

Housed in a 100 percent silicone and waterproof design, INA WAVE offers ten patterns with adjustable speeds. If rabbits aren't your thing, LELO offers the same curling back and forth motion but without the external clitoral stimulator with its Mona Wave G-spot massager.

IROHA MIKAZUKI & MINAMO BY TENGA

2014
Body-safe silicone, ABS plastic
iroha-tenga.com

The first elongated vibrators
from Tenga's iroha brand,
Mikazuki and Minamo have a
pliable design made to fit the
contours of the female body
gently. Created for beginners,
Mikazuki has a thin, crescent-
shaped design, while Minamo
is slightly thicker and features
a rippled edge for increased
sensations.

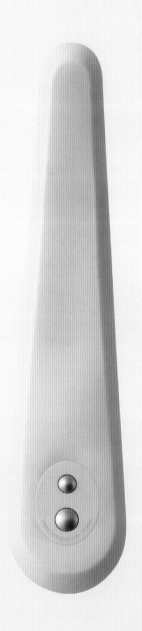

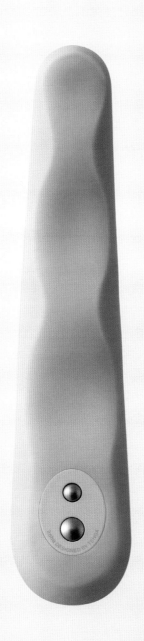

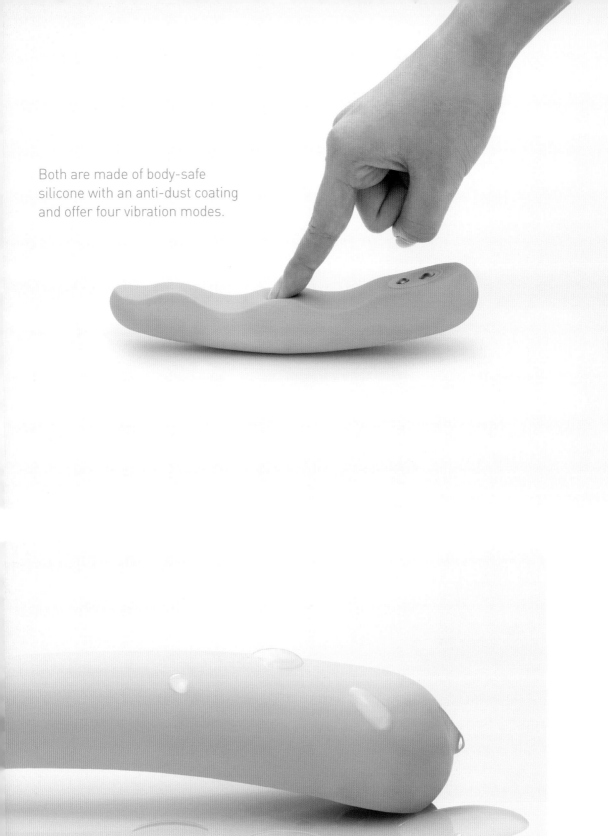

Both are made of body-safe silicone with an anti-dust coating and offer four vibration modes.

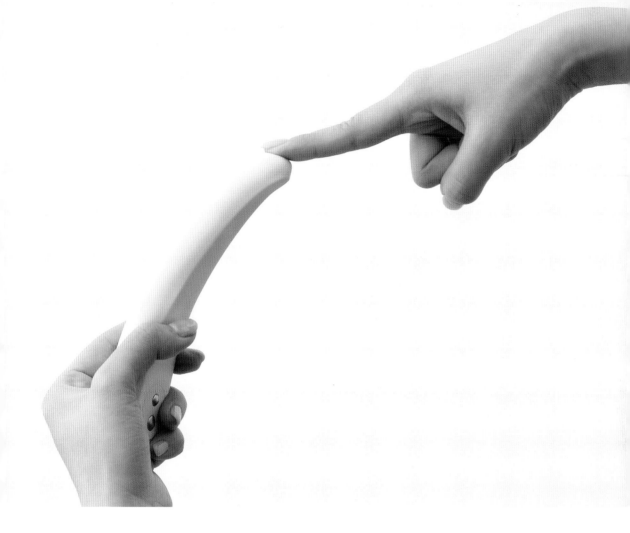

The rechargeable, water-resistant vibes also come with a storage and charging case with an external LED indicator light, making it easier to keep them hidden in plain sight, even while charging.

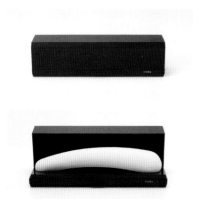

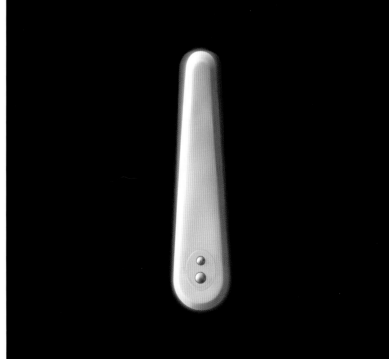

EVA
BY DAME PRODUCTS

2014
Medical-grade silicone, nylon core
dameproducts.com

When Dame Products co-founders and CEOs
Janet Lieberman and Alexandra Fine surpassed
their initial crowdfunding goal for the Eva couples
vibrator in 2014 by over a half-million dollars, they
came one step closer to closing the "pleasure
gap" created by the 70 percent of women who
need clitoral stimulation in order to reach orgasm,
but don't always get it. The two women (an MIT
engineer and a clinical psychologist, respectively)
were motivated by the notion that vibrators can
be vehicles for both empowerment and sexual
wellness.

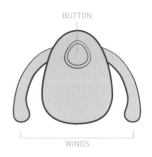

BUTTON

WINGS

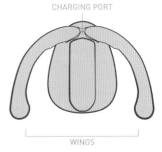

CHARGING PORT

WINGS

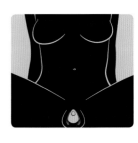

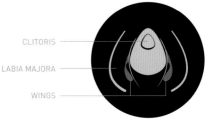

CLITORIS

LABIA MAJORA

WINGS

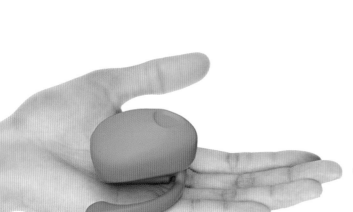

Unlike other hands-free vibes that are inserted into the vagina for added G-spot stimulation, Eva is designed for nonintrusive clitoral stimulation during intercourse. When you first lay eyes on Eva, you half expect this little device to fly away of its own volition. But in fact, those two flexible wings are there to keep this unusual, hands-free, strap-free vibrator securely in place. To insert, put the wings face down towards the vaginal opening, and place the body of the vibe so that it rests on top of the clitoris. The flexible wings are then tucked under the woman's labia majora, where they move with the body. The USB-rechargeable vibe comes with a single button to control three settings, and though it looks like it could swim, it should not be submerged in water.

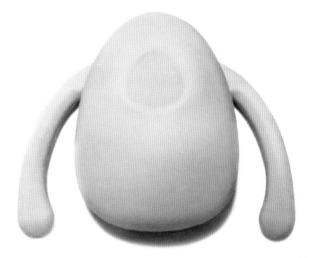

FLEX
BY CRAVE

2015
Silicone, metal
lovecrave.com

As the first company to ever crowdfund
a vibrator project (see Duet on page 84),
Crave is a firm believer in the platform's
ability to build direct relationships with
their customers.

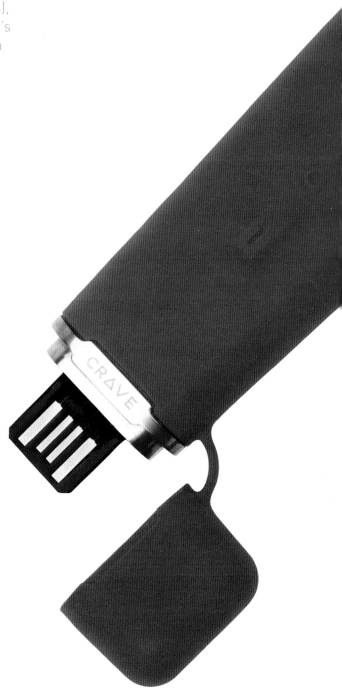

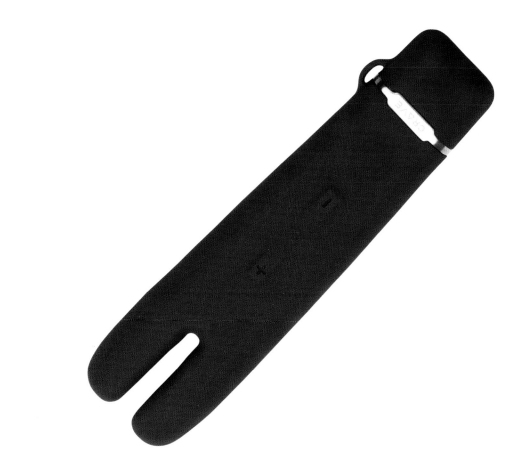

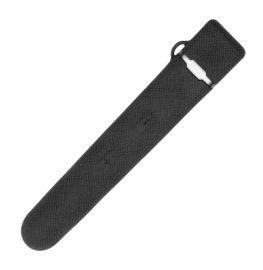

In 2015, the San Francisco-based company held a crowdsourcing project to aggregate data from the first 100 Flex programmable vibrator customers to help them discover which vibration patterns people preferred. It was no easy task, according to the company. Using a statistical method called "k-means," Crave was able to break down the data and divide each pre-defined pattern type into buckets. Each data point submitted was weighted based on the provided rating of that pattern and by any verbal feedback reviewers provided for that pattern.

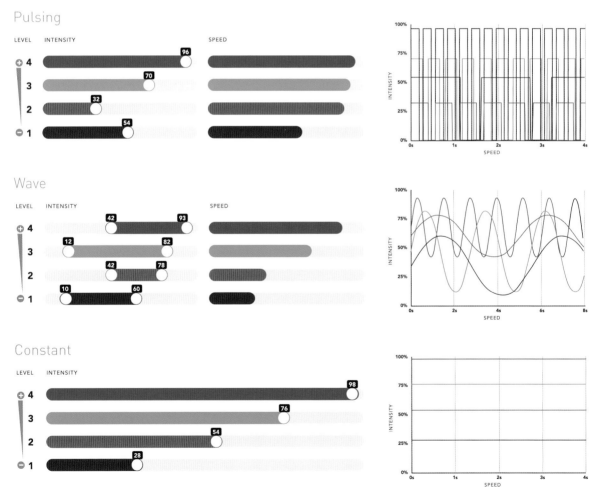

This online interface shows the "greatest hits" selected by customers for the Flex, which includes three modes with four intensities.

After extensive data analysis and number crunching, Crave came up with the "most popular" patterns and intensity settings to bring sixteen of the most desirable vibration patterns to the double-tipped Flex Duet and twelve top patterns to the single-tipped Flex. "It is our hope that these "greatest hits" patterns will better and more fully represent the diverse tastes of the current and future Crave community," says Crave designer Ti Chang. The vibrator comes with unique motor mounts to keep the vibration at the bendy, silicone tips and not in the hand. It charges fully in under two hours via a standard USB port.

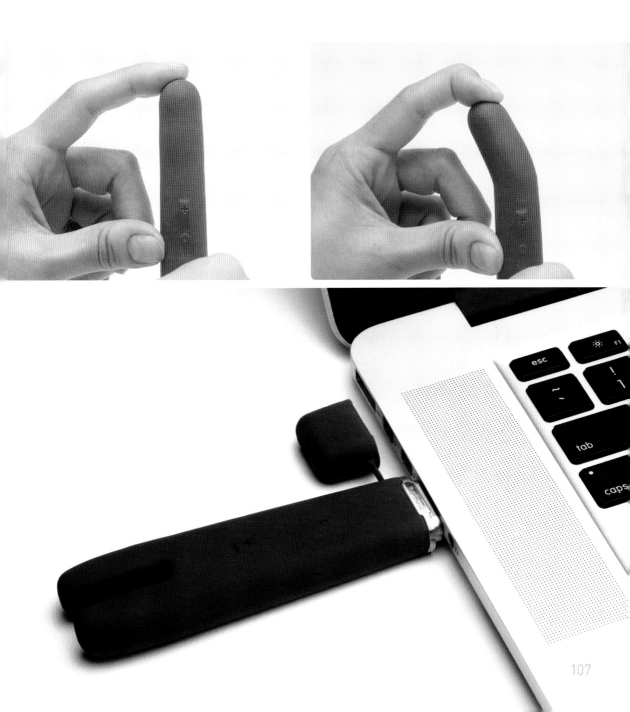

WHOOP.DE.DOO
BY WHOOP.DE.DOO

2015
Medical-grade silicone
whoopdedoo.me

Award-winning industrial designer
Anna Maresova originally developed
the Whoop.de.doo line of erotic toys
as her thesis project at the Faculty
of Art and Design of J. E. Purkyne
University in the Czech Republic
in 2011. Two years later, using her
own savings and a student loan,
the designer launched her brand
with Venus Balls—kegel exercisers
that use a "balls within balls"
mechanism concealed under a
layer of silicone to help strengthen
the pelvic wall.

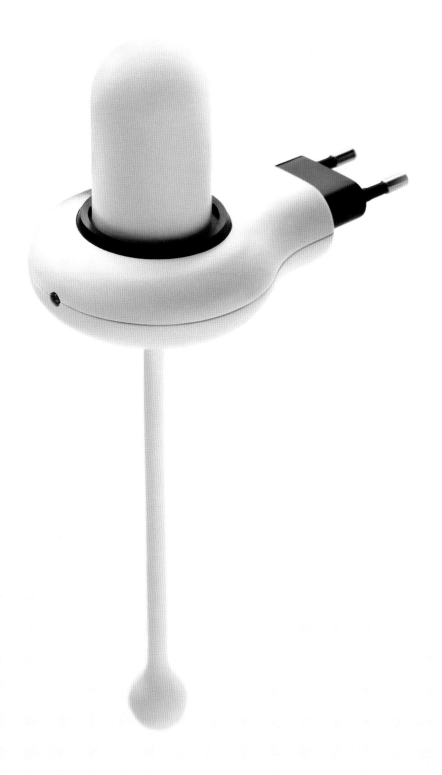

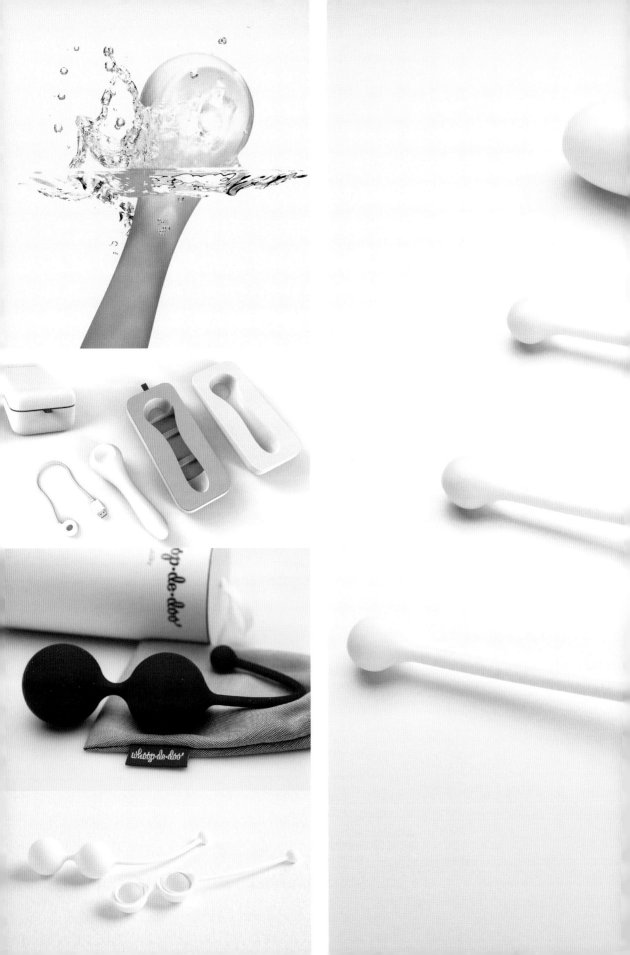

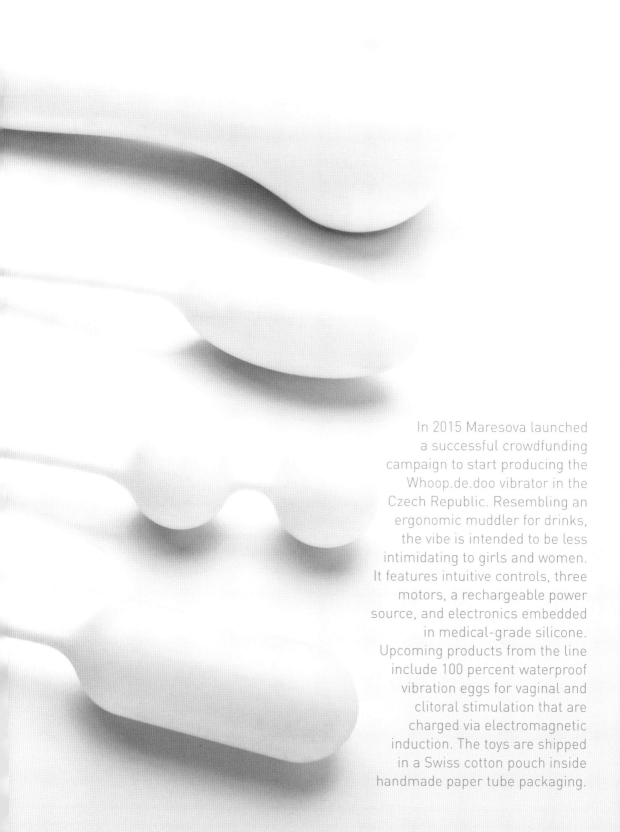

In 2015 Maresova launched a successful crowdfunding campaign to start producing the Whoop.de.doo vibrator in the Czech Republic. Resembling an ergonomic muddler for drinks, the vibe is intended to be less intimidating to girls and women. It features intuitive controls, three motors, a rechargeable power source, and electronics embedded in medical-grade silicone. Upcoming products from the line include 100 percent waterproof vibration eggs for vaginal and clitoral stimulation that are charged via electromagnetic induction. The toys are shipped in a Swiss cotton pouch inside handmade paper tube packaging.

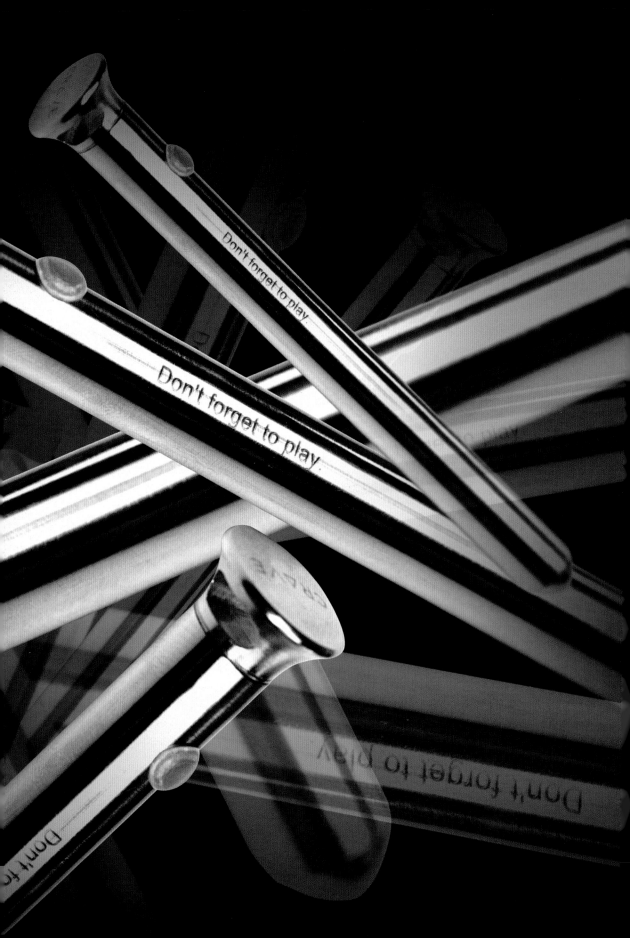

FASHION
& JEWELRY

VESPER
BY CRAVE

2014
Stainless steel, optional 24k gold plating
lovecrave.com

This elegant stainless-steel
pendant has a secret, but its
owners don't have to share it
unless they want to. Designed
by Crave founder Ti Chang,
Vesper is a whisper-quiet but
powerful vibrator for external
stimulation that is worn like a
piece of jewelry. Designed to
hang low on the décolletage,
the Red Dot Award–winning
vibe has a single control button
that can be easily concealed
when worn towards the body.

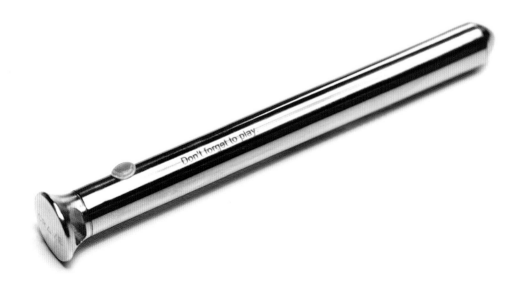

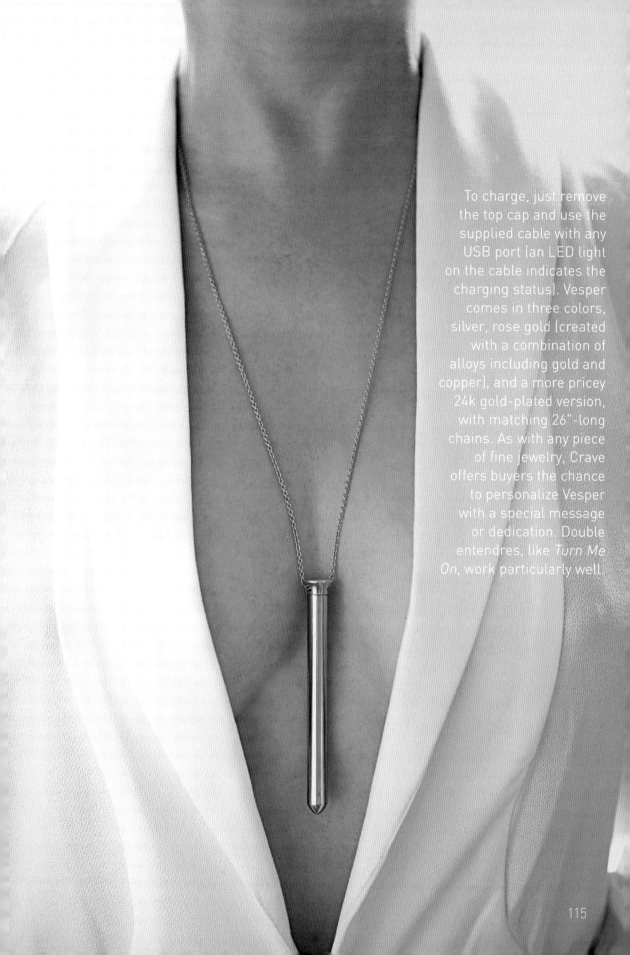

To charge, just remove the top cap and use the supplied cable with any USB port (an LED light on the cable indicates the charging status). Vesper comes in three colors, silver, rose gold (created with a combination of alloys including gold and copper), and a more pricey 24k gold-plated version, with matching 26"-long chains. As with any piece of fine jewelry, Crave offers buyers the chance to personalize Vesper with a special message or dedication. Double entendres, like *Turn Me On*, work particularly well.

DROPLET
BY CRAVE

2009
Stainless steel, sterling silver,
nickel-free electroplated metal base
lovecrave.com

Part of a group of "foreplay
jewelry" designed by Ti
Chang for Crave, the Droplet
features a stainless-steel
silver chain that suspends two
small sterling silver pendant
vibrators. To transform Droplet
into a discreet nipple vibe, just
twist the bottom caps on each
pendant and two quiet motors
deliver a medium-intensity
vibration along the leather loops
that encircle each nipple. Using
four LR48 button cell batteries,
Droplet offers a runtime of ten
to thirty minutes, depending on
the frequency of use.

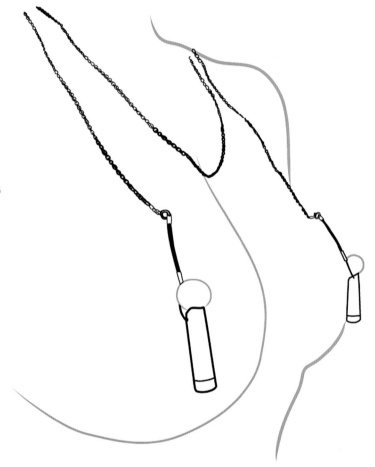

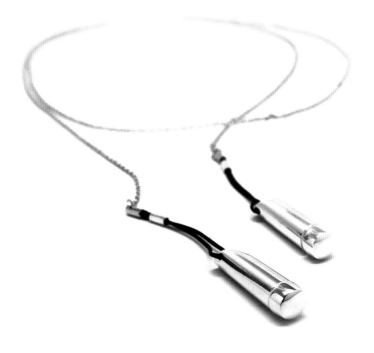

Q&A
TI CHANG
DESIGNER & CO-FOUNDER
CRAVE

Are there any unique challenges or benefits to being a female industrial designer in the sex toy design world?
In any field being a female designer is a challenge. I believe at the same time it is greatly beneficial to have representation of both sexes in the design of products. Specifically in the sex toy industry, where it has been heavily dominated by the male's perspective of what women want, it is so necessary to have trained women designers not just in the conversation, but leading the conversation.

Just because a woman has a clitoris it doesn't mean she can proxy the market for all women. A sex toy that works for one person may not be a fit for another, and that's just how it goes. Clitorises come in all different shapes and sizes, so I think being a good designer is most important. Whether a man or woman, it's important not just to be able to listen and work well with the aesthetic of the product but to be able to work fluidly with a team of engineers, manufacturers, and researchers to design and produce the highest-quality product possible.

Are there many women designers in this industry?
There are many women behind companies and they are very much the backbone of the industry and part of the product development process of a sex toy, but very few are actually trained industrial designers. And that really makes a difference when it comes to the design of the product. Industrial designers are not just about how a product looks. They also understand user-centered research informs the design, and with their understanding of manufacturing, the product really comes to life. Having this holistic view is important to designing more modern products.

How did you get started designing objects of pleasure?
I got started designing sex toys when I realized it was a category of products that needed to be revamped. I remember seeing the sea of hot pink dildos and flesh-colored penises and I thought why can't sex toys be just as elevated and well made as a mobile phone or any other electronic consumer product?

So I started Incognito designing wearable jewelry meets discreet sex toys. I wanted to elevate the idea of what we would normally think of as sex toys and break the preconceived notion of traditional sex toys in a fashionable way. The idea of adornment, such as jewelry pieces, transformed into a toy intrigued me.

My first design was actually a pair of double bracelets that can be used as cuffs for restraint. It seemed so obvious that bracelets should be able to be used for that . . . to me anyway.

How do you see sex toys evolving in the next decade?
I think the conversation about sex and sex toys will shift dramatically in the next decade. I am hopeful for the better: better in terms of openness, as-matter-of-factly, without shame and stigma. With this major shift in cultural attitude and more advanced technology I can't even begin to imagine the amazing products/experiences that will be created.

What kind of feedback (positive or negative) do you get when talking to customers about typical sex toys?
Sometimes it can be difficult for customers to tell you exactly what they want. Often it's easier for them to tell you what they don't want. It is not a mystery that most find the current "standard" sex toys ridiculous in terms of the colors, shapes, motifs, and quality.

Which sex toy product type do you think is in most need of a redesign?
The life-like silicone body parts, like torsos, vaginas, and butts . . . there has got to be a less . . . realistic solution.

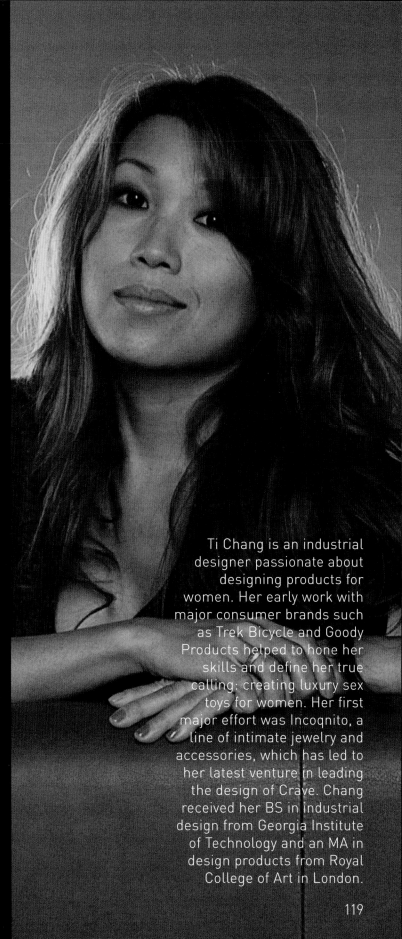

Is the stigma related
to sex toys improving?
Oh absolutely, you can now buy
a vibrator at a Walgreens and
at Brookstone at the mall—
that's pretty mainstream. Our
product Duet is the world's first
crowdfunded sex toy—we were
trying to raise $15K and we ended
up meeting that in 48 hours and
raising over $100,000. These are
pretty clear indicators that as a
society, we feel less taboo about
sex toys than we have in the past.

The stigma that kept people away
from the industry is changing
so rapidly and becoming
mainstream. As long as a
designer doesn't have a negative
attitude towards sex toys there is
nothing strange or different about
designing sex toys vs. a camera.
The design process is the same.

Ti Chang is an industrial
designer passionate about
designing products for
women. Her early work with
major consumer brands such
as Trek Bicycle and Goody
Products helped to hone her
skills and define her true
calling: creating luxury sex
toys for women. Her first
major effort was Incoqnito, a
line of intimate jewelry and
accessories, which has led to
her latest venture in leading
the design of Crave. Chang
received her BS in industrial
design from Georgia Institute
of Technology and an MA in
design products from Royal
College of Art in London.

LEATHER TASSELS BY CRAVE

2009
Leather, stainless steel
lovecrave.com

Like little bolo ties for the breasts, these adjustable,
lightweight tassels were designed by Ti Chang of
Crave to fit around most nipple sizes. The tassels
are crafted of thin genuine leather strings with
stainless-steel metal accents. The tassels—which
can be worn under clothing or put on as part of
foreplay—are a gentler alternative to clamps or
other nipple-stimulation devices.

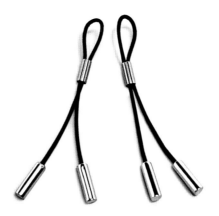

MÉNAGE À QUATRE RINGS
BY VIVIANE YAZDANI

2013
Body-safe silicone, silver
menageaquatre.net

Milan-based designer Viviane Yazdani thinks that
if you like it then you should put a ring on it. While
not quite as adventurous as a *ménage à trois*, this
foursome is designed for female self-pleasure, a
subject that still remains taboo. The rings, which
were presented at an offsite event during the 2014
Salone del Mobile in Milan, were developed by
Yazdani specifically to stimulate the clitoris and
other pleasurable areas of the body.

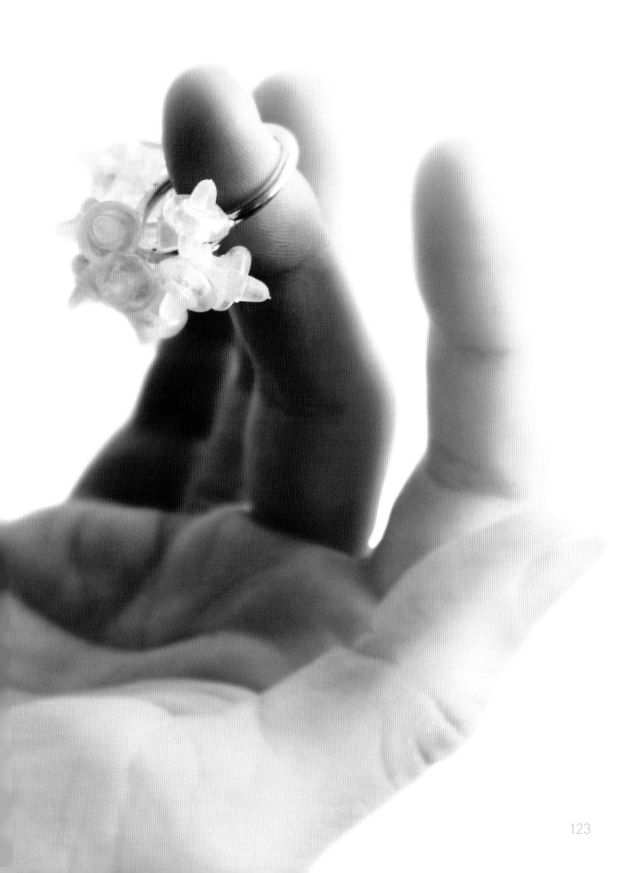

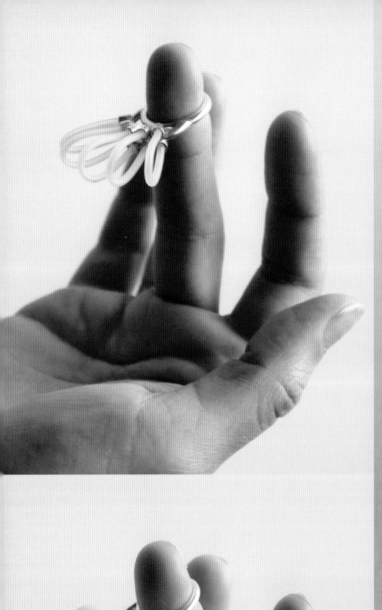

A work in progress, the rings include La Douce (for the sweetest), La Rêveuse (for the dreamers), La Joueuse (for the playful), and La Non-Timide (for the less shy). Each ring has a different set of beads resembling long loops, nipple-like nubs, pearls, or small triangles, to create a unique sensation—from soft to intense. Made of high-grade, body-safe silicone and silver, the rings are waterproof and easy to wash.

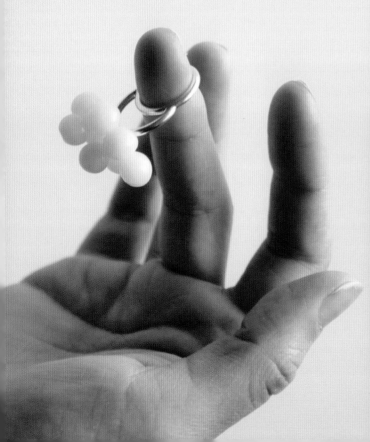

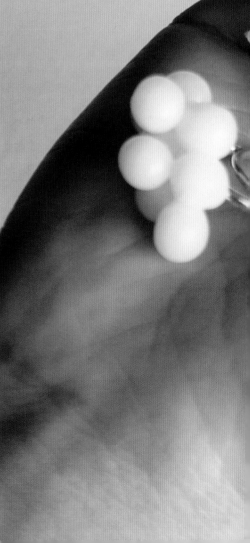

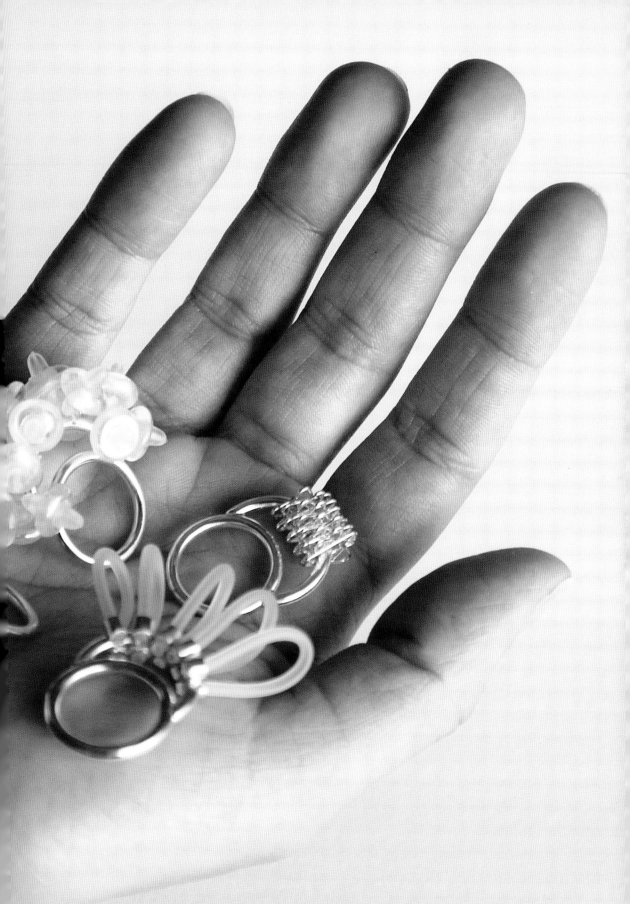

Q&A
BLISS LAU
BODY JEWELRY DESIGNER

Do you feel that your cultural background has influenced your design work at all?
We will always be influenced by our backgrounds. Being internally composed of two different cultures is also parallel to my early life in Hawaii and adult life in New York. The juxtaposition of cultures is absolutely translated into my work; I feel it is the source of my need to make products that have a strong hard/soft balance and consistent flexibility.

Can you tell us how you made the transition from women's handbags to designing body chains?
If only someone could create a definition for the creative process, all of our journeys would be so much easier! My experience as a designer has been through a series of discoveries based on exploration, execution, experience, and then finally consistent change and new discovery.

Handbags were my first exploration. I realized after about four to five years that my love for design was ornamental and not utilitarian. That was the day in 2007 that I designed a full set of body chain concepts and eventually canceled the handbags altogether to focus on tracing lines on the body.

Why did you choose to work with cultured pearls and onyx?
For two years I researched materials for my Fibonacci Sequence and pearls and onyx were chosen because of their opposite origins. Much like my internalized juxtaposition of two cultures, pearls come from the water and rise above to join us, while onyx is born from a volcano. The ideas of black and white, as well as the rich history of the pearl representing perfection, were beautiful parallels to the golden ratio, also being a basis for design.

Which artists and designers inspire your work?
The list is endless. I am inspired by tangibles and intangibles. Anaïs Nin's poetry has inspired many of my sensual lingerie-based body chains such as the Lost in Light bra. Shakespeare inspired the Dark Lady body chain as well as the Fathom ring, which was created after listening to a sonnet from *The Tempest*. Visual artists also inspire me, as well as musicians, from Robert Wilson's light design to Nick Cave or the cellist Maya Beiser.

Do you have any advice for other fashion designers who are interested in experimenting in more sensual designs?
Be fearless, it's the only way to tap into the part of yourself that can create something new.

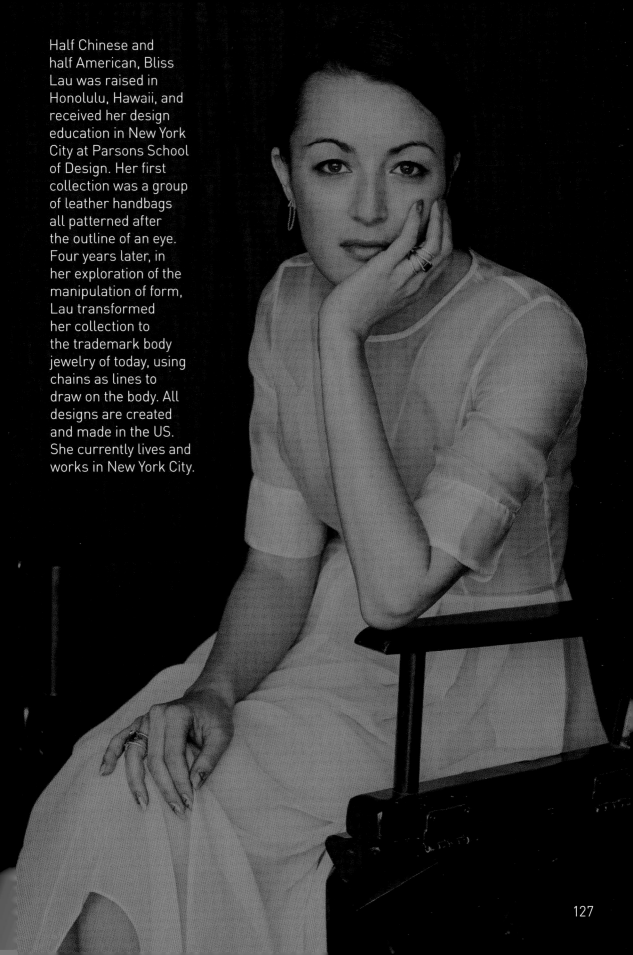

Half Chinese and half American, Bliss Lau was raised in Honolulu, Hawaii, and received her design education in New York City at Parsons School of Design. Her first collection was a group of leather handbags all patterned after the outline of an eye. Four years later, in her exploration of the manipulation of form, Lau transformed her collection to the trademark body jewelry of today, using chains as lines to draw on the body. All designs are created and made in the US. She currently lives and works in New York City.

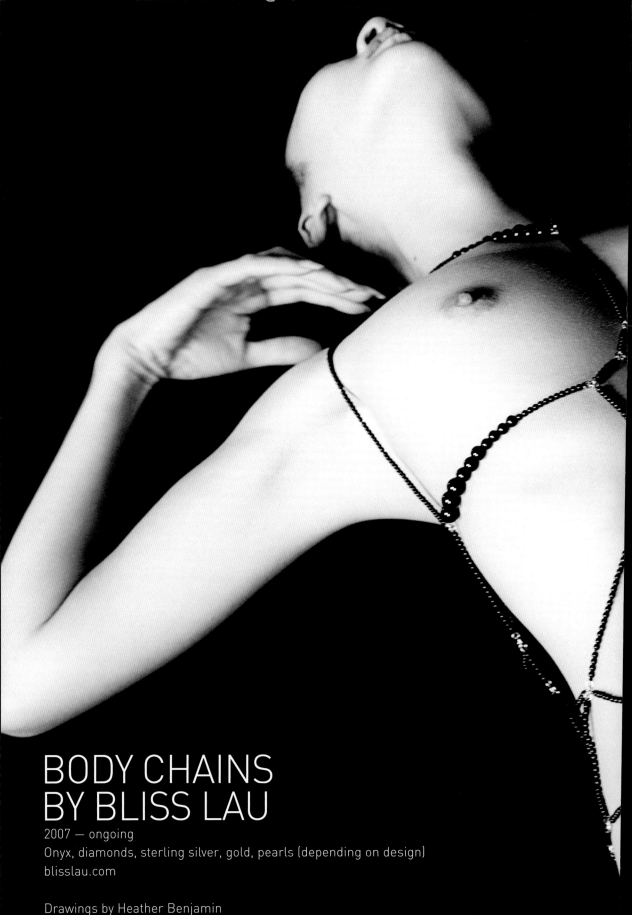

BODY CHAINS
BY BLISS LAU

2007 — ongoing
Onyx, diamonds, sterling silver, gold, pearls (depending on design)
blisslau.com

Drawings by Heather Benjamin

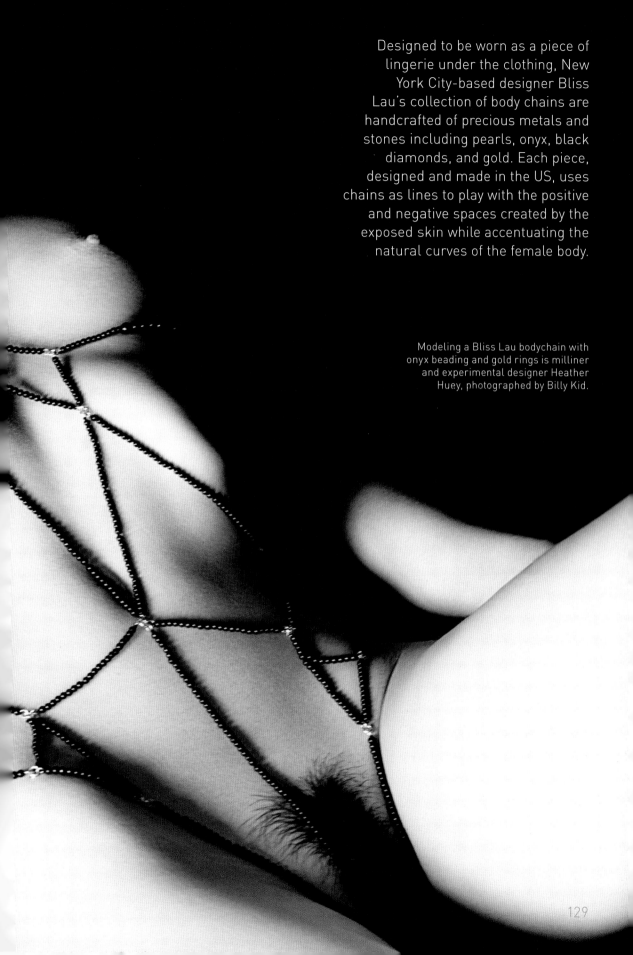

Designed to be worn as a piece of lingerie under the clothing, New York City-based designer Bliss Lau's collection of body chains are handcrafted of precious metals and stones including pearls, onyx, black diamonds, and gold. Each piece, designed and made in the US, uses chains as lines to play with the positive and negative spaces created by the exposed skin while accentuating the natural curves of the female body.

Modeling a Bliss Lau bodychain with onyx beading and gold rings is milliner and experimental designer Heather Huey, photographed by Billy Kid.

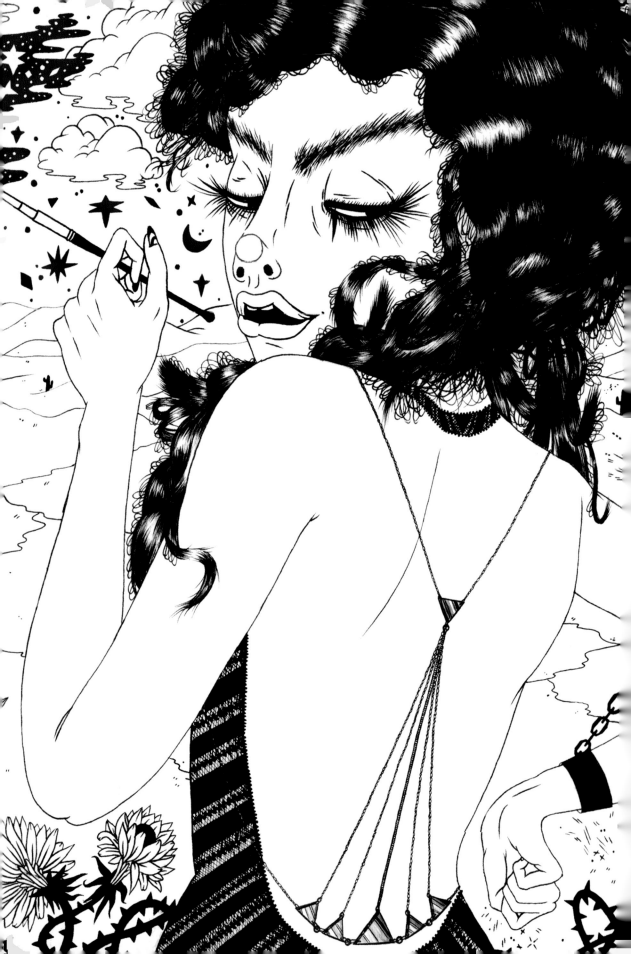

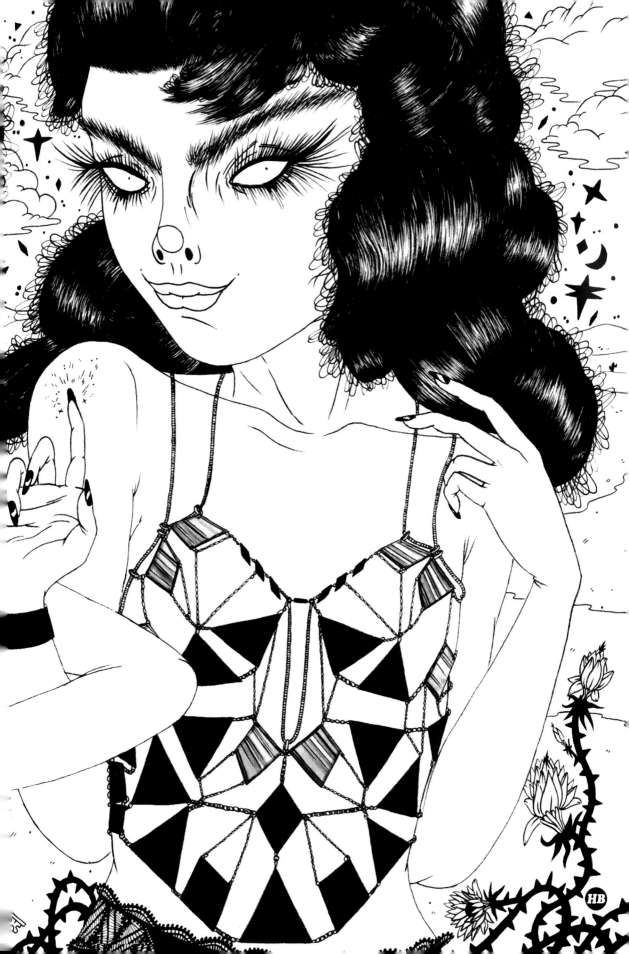

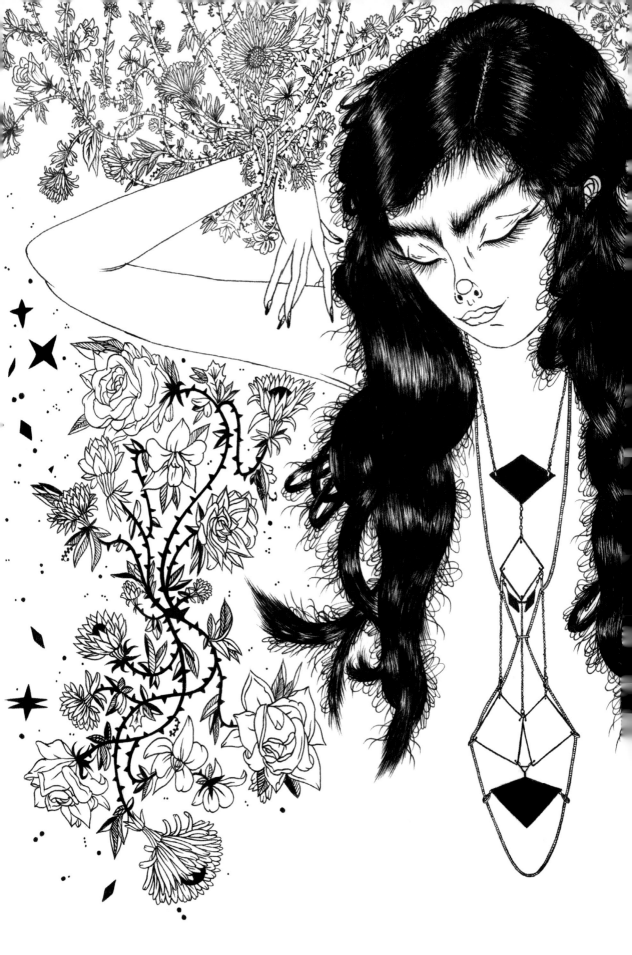

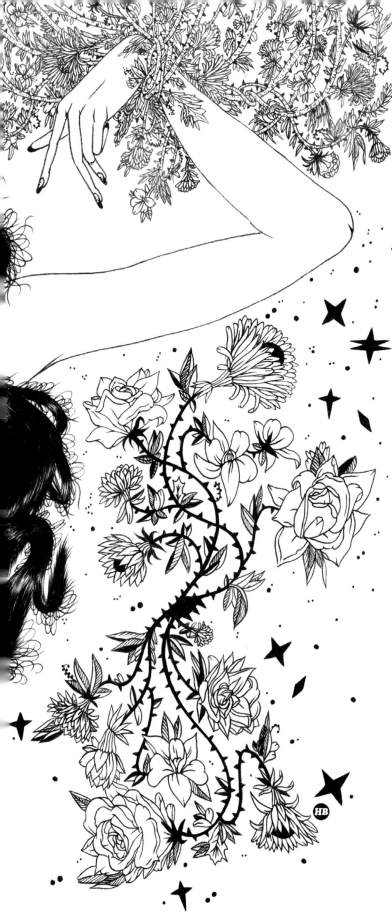

Lau finds inspiration in literature and music, but also science, as seen in her pieces based on the Fibonacci sequence. The designer says she has developed a cult following for women looking for highly specialized and personalized pieces of lingerie. "My client is in touch with her sexuality," explains Lau, "but not in an overt way."

In 2015, Lau created the Love to Love Me limited-edition bodychain exclusively for Kiki De Montparnesse boutiques in New York, Los Angeles, and Las Vegas. Designed to fit almost any body type or shape, the sterling silver chain is adorned with a black diamond and can be worn over the heart or down the spine.

Fantastical drawings by illustrator Heather Benjamin feature Bliss Lau body chains and jewelry (this page and previous spread).

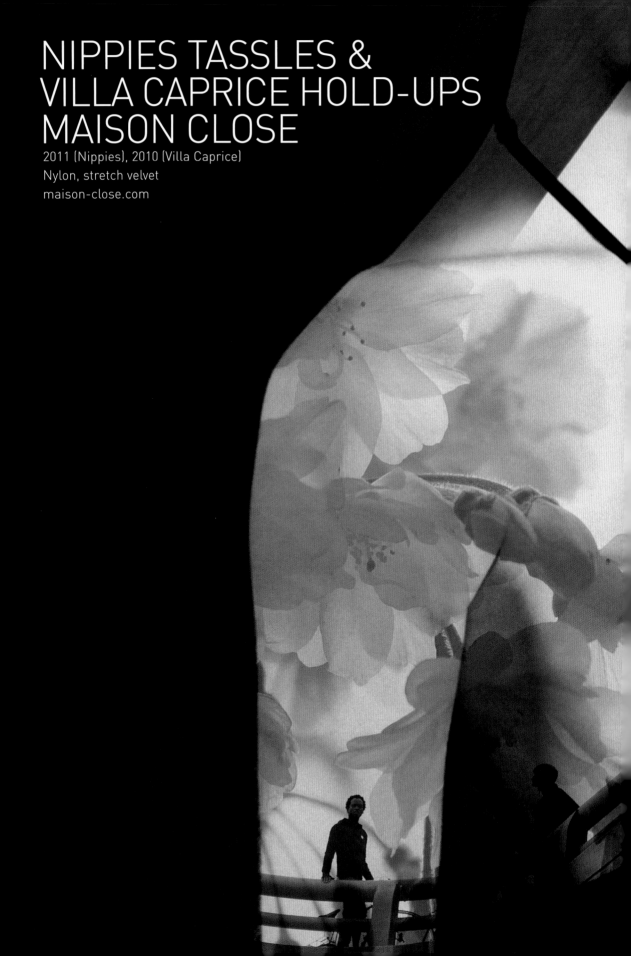

NIPPIES TASSLES &
VILLA CAPRICE HOLD-UPS
MAISON CLOSE

2011 (Nippies), 2010 (Villa Caprice)
Nylon, stretch velvet
maison-close.com

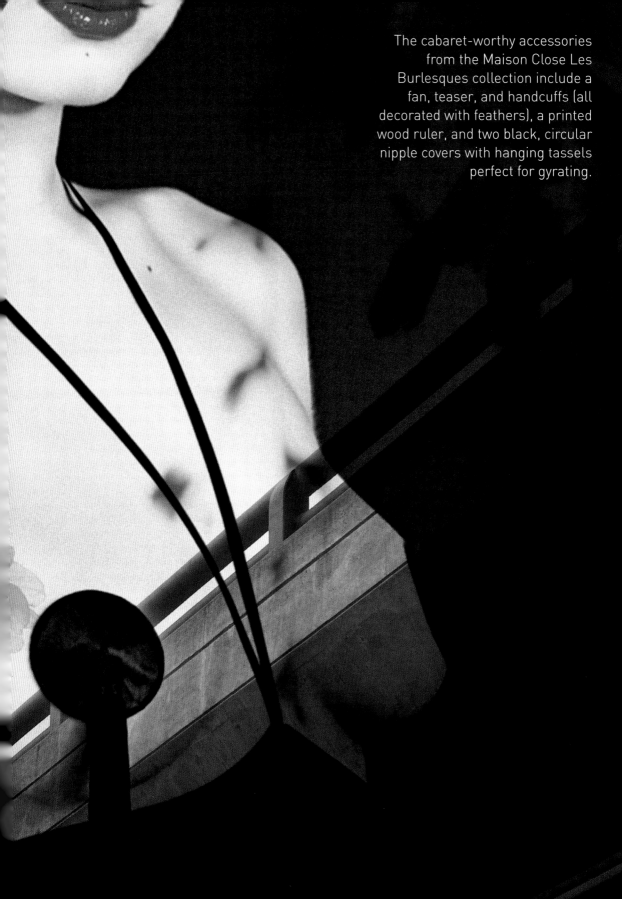

The cabaret-worthy accessories from the Maison Close Les Burlesques collection include a fan, teaser, and handcuffs (all decorated with feathers), a printed wood ruler, and two black, circular nipple covers with hanging tassels perfect for gyrating.

Also fit for the stage are the Villa Caprice line from the brand's Les Fétiches collection. Villa Caprice includes two leg hold-ups, two arm coverings, and a body-hugging belt all in black, velvet elastic to help keep them in place. Like all Maison Close products, these pieces are designed in-house by brand creator Nicolas Busnel.

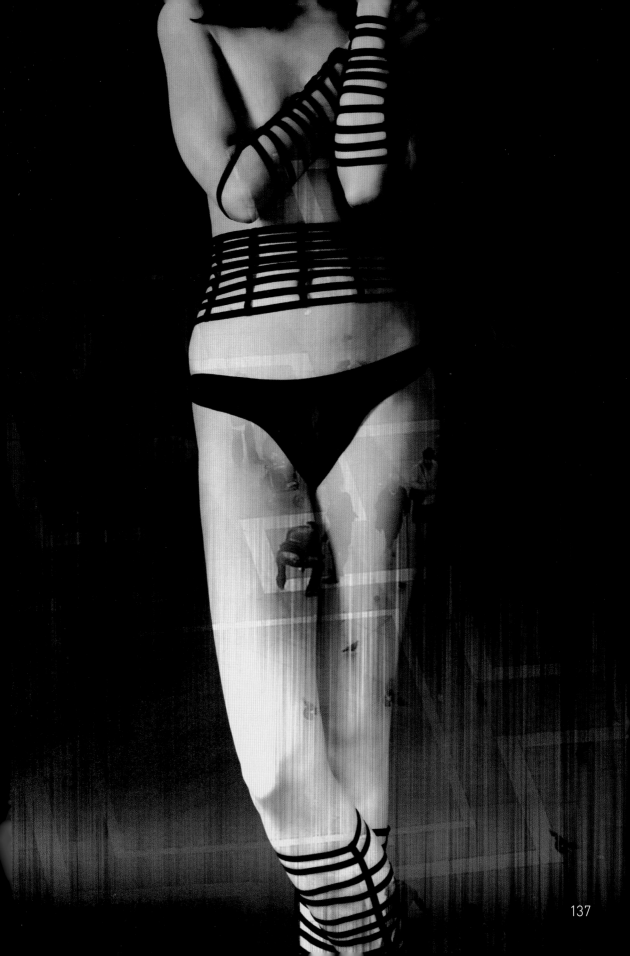

REVOLUTIONARY LINGERIE COLLECTION & PASTIES BY WONDERPUSS OCTOPUS

2014 (Revolutionary Collection), 2013 (Pasties)
Silicone, latex, dimensional fabric paint
wonderpussoctopusink.com

Wonderpuss Octopus, a.k.a. the Brooklyn-based artist PJ Linden, explores "texture fetishism" with her incredibly detailed, multilayered strata of 3D fabric paint, acrylic, and latex. "I pull from beading traditions and patterns found in nature, especially aquatic life," says Linden, who likes to juxtapose her designs with pop culture items like candy sprinkles.

Linden began refining her trademark "bubbling" paint technique (a.k.a. 3D fabric paint or puffy paint) back in 2005 in order to find her voice as an artist. By layering the material, which she describes as liquid plastic, Linden sculpts "second skins" for everyday objects like cameras and sneakers, or more intimate items like pasties, anal beads, and butt plugs. "I became fascinated with the preservation possibilities," says Linden. "I began encasing not only canvas and wood panels but also ready-mades of our time: technology, luxury goods, and modern tools. In a way, my work becomes this sarcophagus, this plastic shield."

The 3D fabric paint offers several benefits, including a greater lifespan than oil paint and the ability to be submerged in water and heated to very high temperatures. Although Linden painstakingly hand-paints each piece, the patterns are so precise that people assume the work is machine made. Shown here are a few of Linden's wearable art pieces, including the Magic Pelt bra, balaclava, and handcuffs, and the Starfish, Flower Pearl, and Ivory Urchin Pasties.

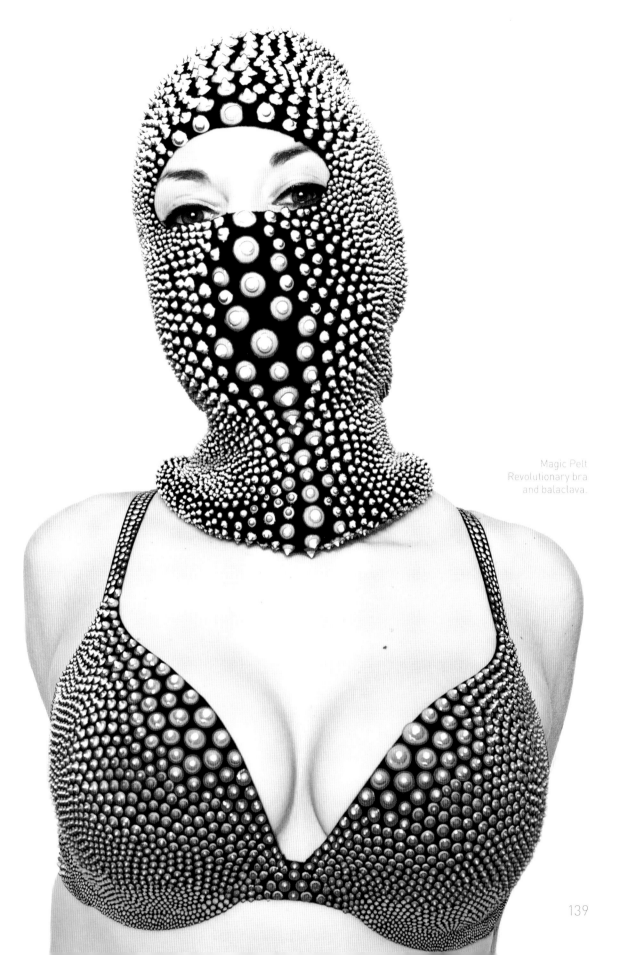

Magic Pelt
Revolutionary bra
and balaclava.

139

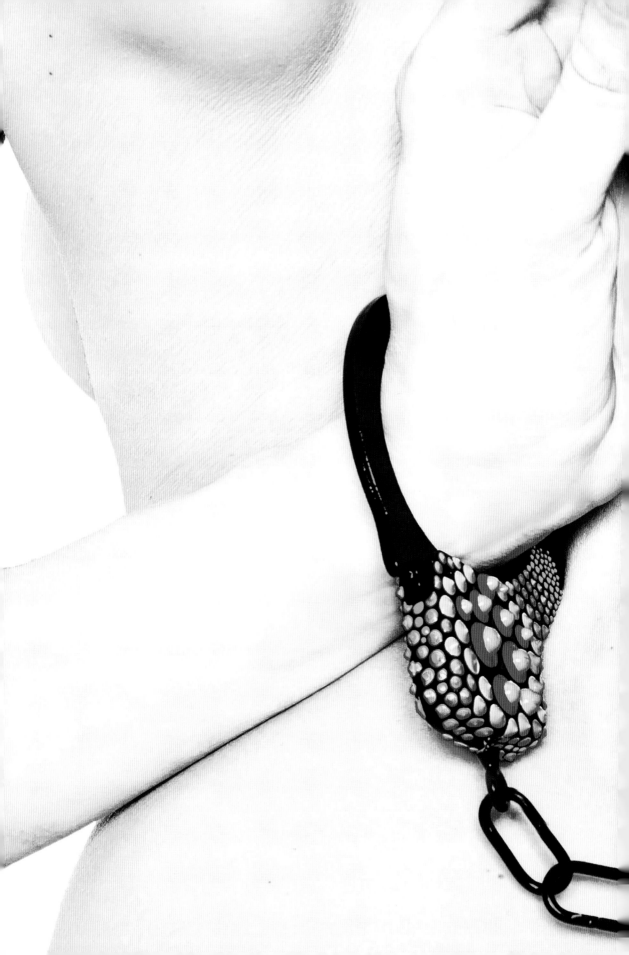

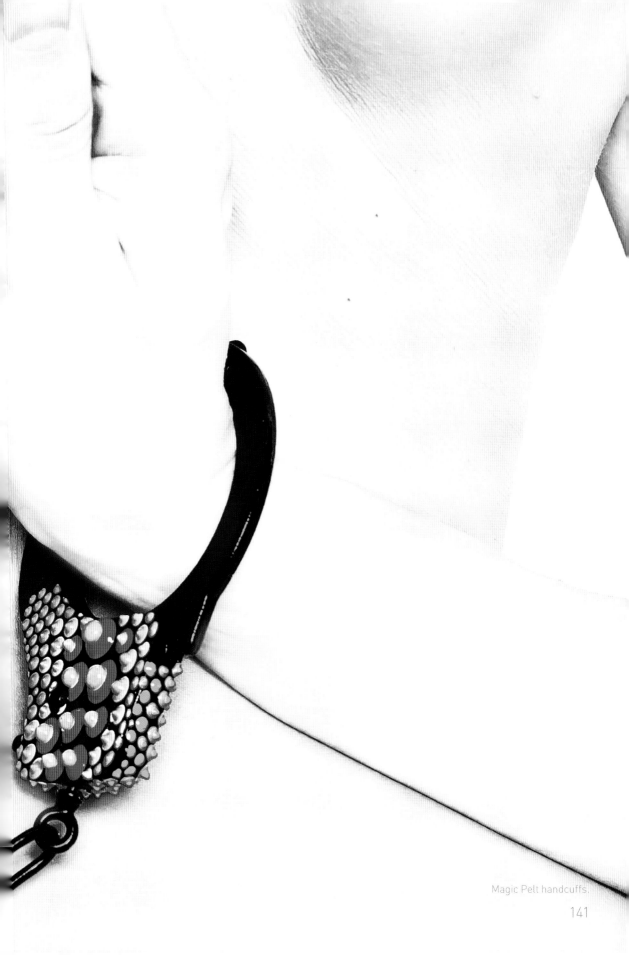

Magic Pelt handcuffs.

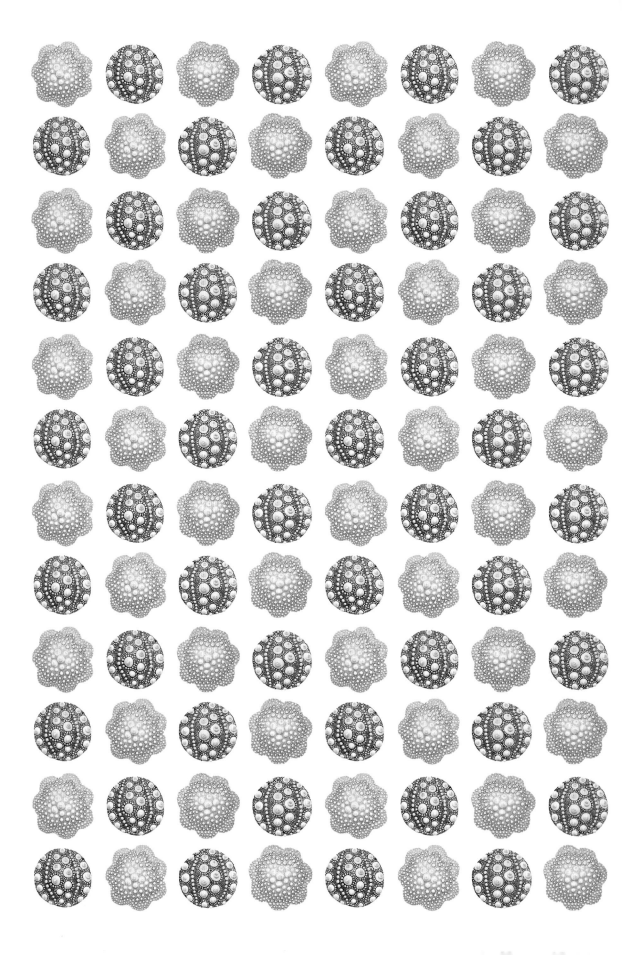

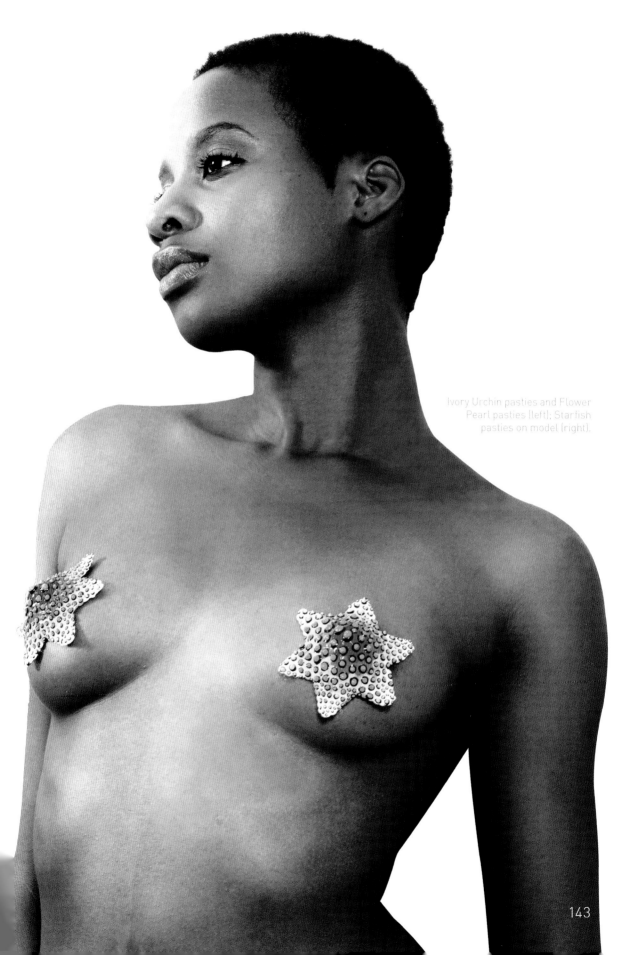

Ivory Urchin pasties and Flower
Pearl pasties (left); Starfish
pasties on model (right).

YOURETHRA COCK PIN & CROSS NIP NIPPLE JEWELRY BY ROSEBUDS

1997 (Yourethra), 1996 (Cross Nip)
Medical-grade stainless steel, bronze
rosebuds.net

Best known for its line of bejeweled butt plugs, the French sex toy company Rosebuds also makes jewelry to adorn the nipples, penis, or scrotum. Not for the faint of heart, the 2.75"-long Yourethra cock pin "ornaments your sex like a champagne cork," according to the manufacturer. To use, the stainless-steel urethral stem is lubricated before it is inserted into the urethra of the penis. A bronze ring held in place by four silver chains further increases pressure to the area.

For less invasive play, Cross Nip is a pair of brass jewels that create a very tight framing of the nipples, giving them the illusion of being pierced. Gently turning the square-shaped brass clips increases sensation. Both pieces are designed by Rosebuds's late founder Julian Snelling, the creator of the original Swarovski-encrusted Rosebud butt plug in 1996.

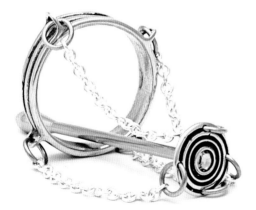

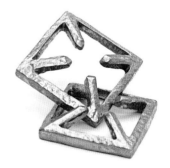

LATEX COUTURE APPAREL BY DAWNAMATRIX

2009 – ongoing
Latex, canvas, hardware, boning
dawnamatrix.com

After living in Japan for several years, fashion designer Dawn Mostow wanted to establish a latex clothing company based on the principles of fine art. She relocated to New York City, where she earned a master of fine arts from Pratt Institute and refined her clothing design skills working on theatrical costume design for opera.

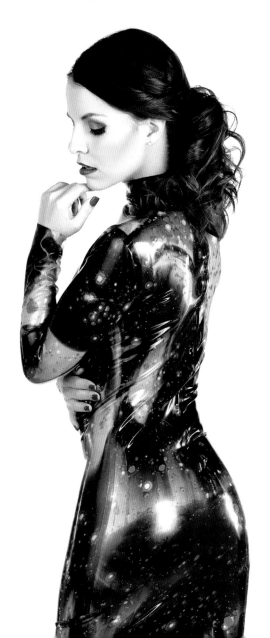

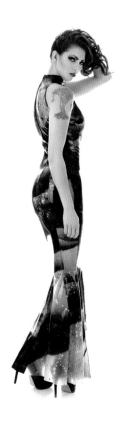

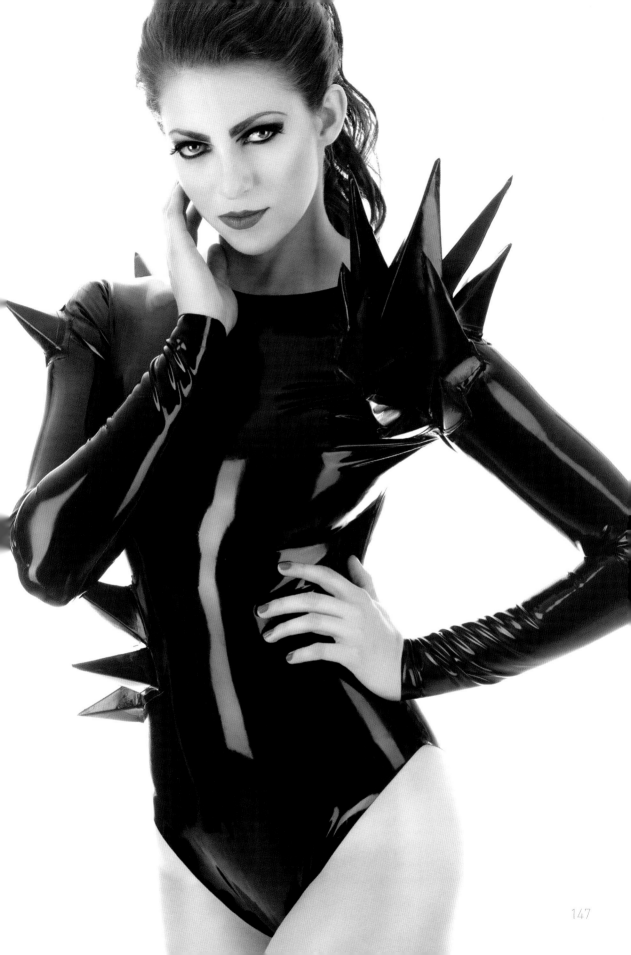

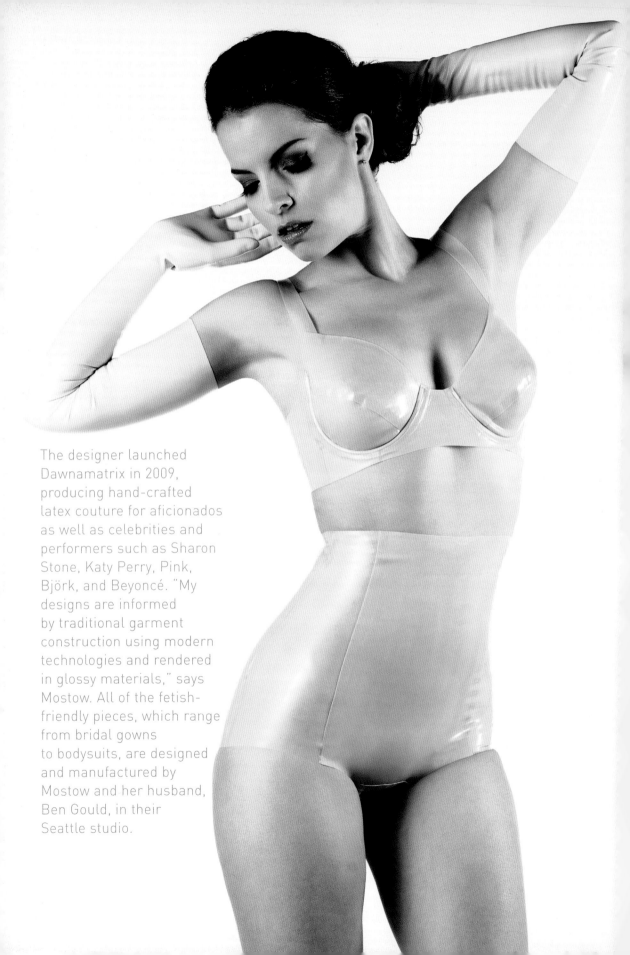

The designer launched Dawnamatrix in 2009, producing hand-crafted latex couture for aficionados as well as celebrities and performers such as Sharon Stone, Katy Perry, Pink, Björk, and Beyoncé. "My designs are informed by traditional garment construction using modern technologies and rendered in glossy materials," says Mostow. All of the fetish-friendly pieces, which range from bridal gowns to bodysuits, are designed and manufactured by Mostow and her husband, Ben Gould, in their Seattle studio.

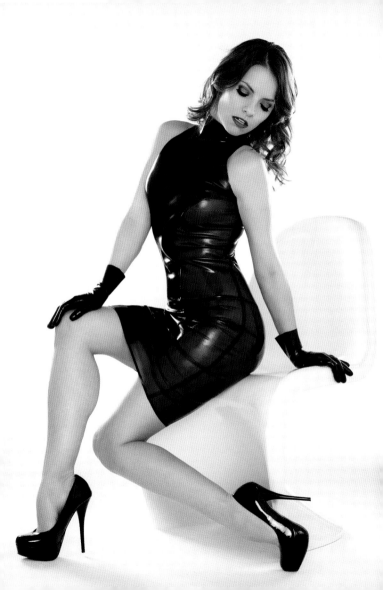

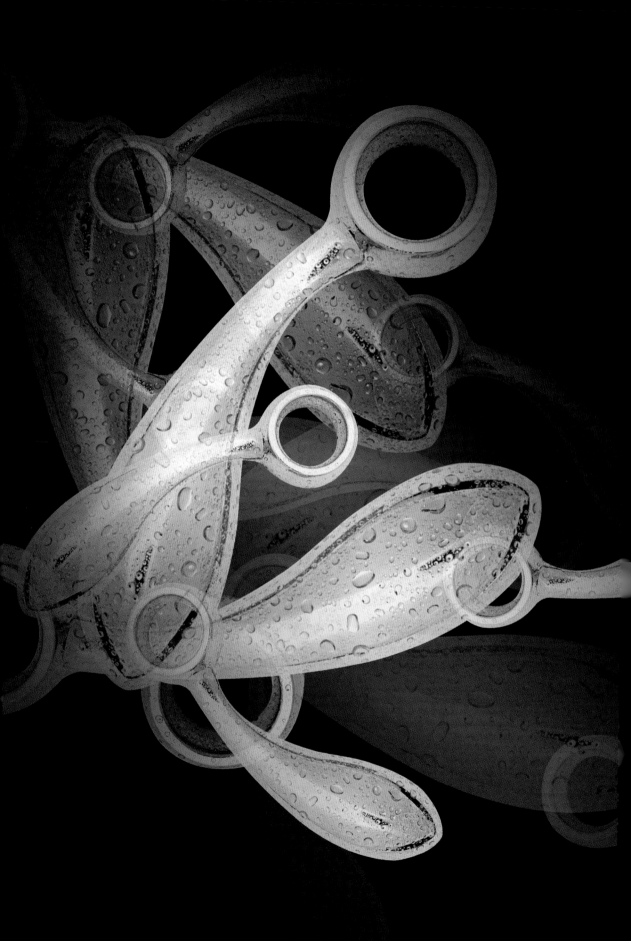

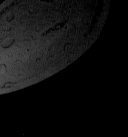

COCK RINGS & ANAL TOYS

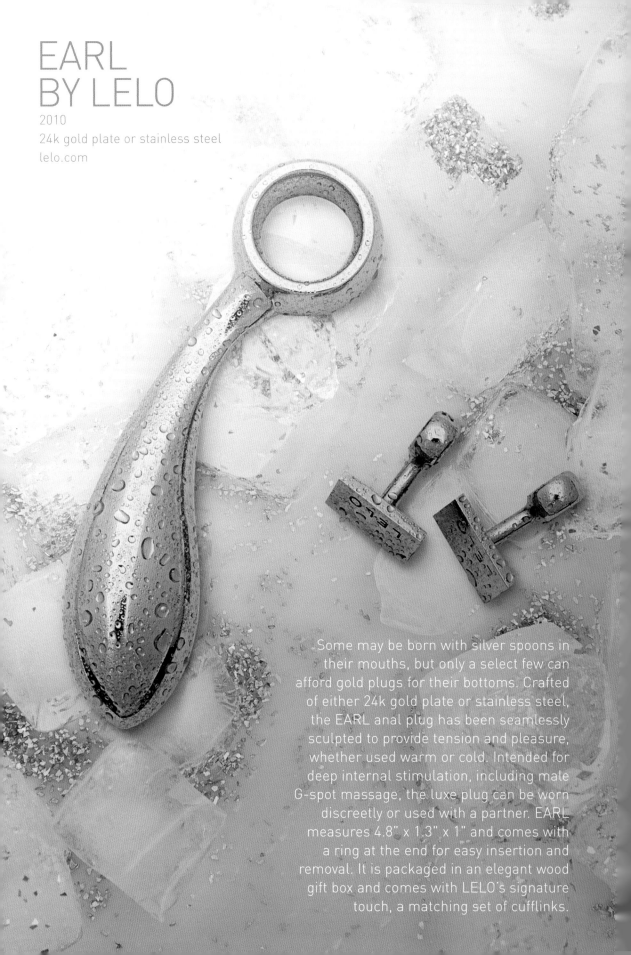

EARL
BY LELO

2010
24k gold plate or stainless steel
lelo.com

Some may be born with silver spoons in their mouths, but only a select few can afford gold plugs for their bottoms. Crafted of either 24k gold plate or stainless steel, the EARL anal plug has been seamlessly sculpted to provide tension and pleasure, whether used warm or cold. Intended for deep internal stimulation, including male G-spot massage, the luxe plug can be worn discreetly or used with a partner. EARL measures 4.8" x 1.3" x 1" and comes with a ring at the end for easy insertion and removal. It is packaged in an elegant wood gift box and comes with LELO's signature touch, a matching set of cufflinks.

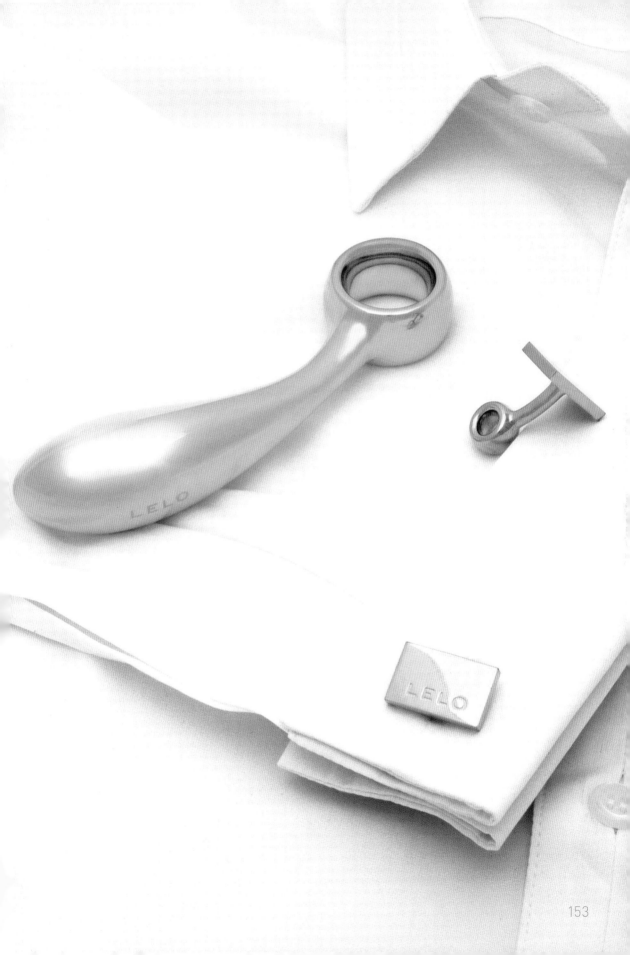

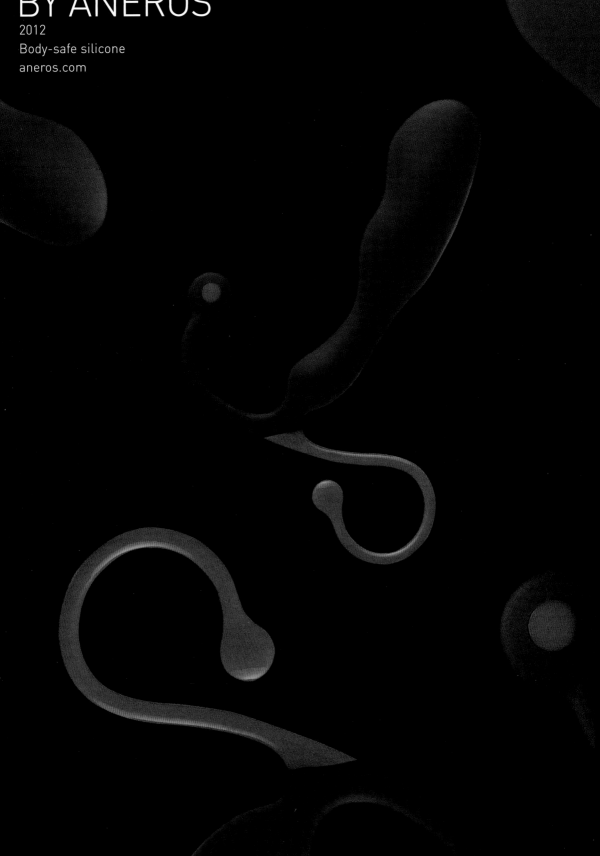

HELIXSYN
BY ANEROS

2012

Body-safe silicone

aneros.com

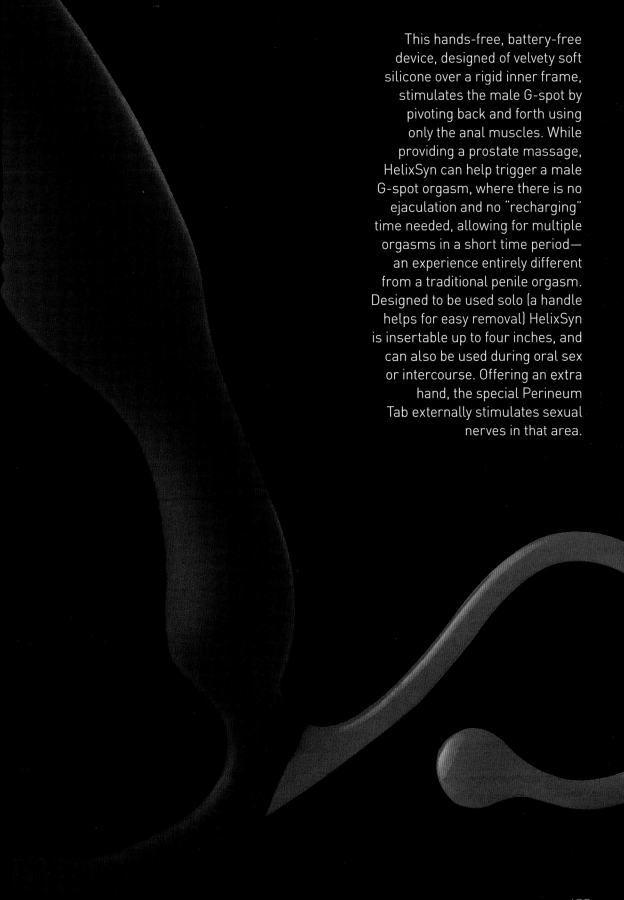

This hands-free, battery-free device, designed of velvety soft silicone over a rigid inner frame, stimulates the male G-spot by pivoting back and forth using only the anal muscles. While providing a prostate massage, HelixSyn can help trigger a male G-spot orgasm, where there is no ejaculation and no "recharging" time needed, allowing for multiple orgasms in a short time period—an experience entirely different from a traditional penile orgasm. Designed to be used solo (a handle helps for easy removal) HelixSyn is insertable up to four inches, and can also be used during oral sex or intercourse. Offering an extra hand, the special Perineum Tab externally stimulates sexual nerves in that area.

Q&A
EPIPHORA
SEX BLOGGER

HeyEpiphora.com

Which sex toy type do you feel has improved the most since you began reviewing? Which needs a design overhaul?
Small rechargeable clitoral vibrators have really taken off. There were a few already in circulation when I started reviewing in 2007, but a bunch have come out since, from companies such as LELO, Je Joue, We-Vibe, and Jimmyjane. Rechargeable toys in general have become a lot more commonplace, with even the larger, old school companies releasing some. I approve of this trend!

I think we have some work to do on toys for penises. When it comes to both cock rings and sleeves, a lot of the toys are still made of porous materials, so they're difficult to clean and can't be shared. I also would love to see more vibrators for penises.

Do you think that sex toys have become more mainstream in recent years or do they still have a fair degree of stigma attached to them?
They've had their moments, for sure. When they get mainstream attention, they're less stigmatized for a while. But I think after the excitement wears off, and without that icebreaker question ("Have you read *Fifty Shades of Grey*?", "Did you see that *Sex and the City* episode?"), people go right back to being hush-hush about sex toys.

Several myths persist: that sex toys are addictive, numbing, only for lonely people. It'll be quite a while before the public regards sex toys with the same affection that I do.

You have an impressive collection of toys. How do you store them? Which ones do you choose to display and which do you choose to keep private?
I keep them in several chests of plastic drawers. I have one chest for chargers and batteries, and four more for the toys themselves. I display a couple Vixen Creations dildos on the shelf above my computer, because they must be stored upright (and because they are neon green and tie dye!). I also have some adorable miniature dildos that live on that shelf, along with a framed knitted vulva.

Is there ever a toy that is appealing from a product design angle that fails to impress when you test it out? On the other hand, are there products that look terribly designed but then knock it out of the park?
Absolutely. The word "revolutionary" is trotted out a lot these days, often alongside a promise of innovative new technology. There's a spherical toy that uses sonic technology to move a piston back and forth. The problem is, the piston doesn't deliver enough strength to be stimulating on most settings. Another toy claims to move "like a finger," but it only has one speed and it was so loud I couldn't hear myself think.

Usually if something looks really badly designed, it is. What really surprises me are the toys that seem too simple, but end up becoming my favorites. The LELO Mona 2 is a great example of this. Although the design does not appear to be spectacular, I was won over by the ergonomic shape, ease of use, and range of vibration intensities.

What advice would you give a young product designer looking to enter the sex toy design world?
Do your research and get to know the industry. If you think that all sex toys are toxic, take a moment to familiarize yourself with all the wonderful companies that produce body-safe toys (and have been for ten years). Be willing to listen, especially if you don't have a vagina of your own. Test your toys in advance on discerning genitals. When you release a product, don't act like the sex toy industry's savior, and don't use bombastic language like "the world's first." Focus on what makes your design different, yes, but be humble about it.

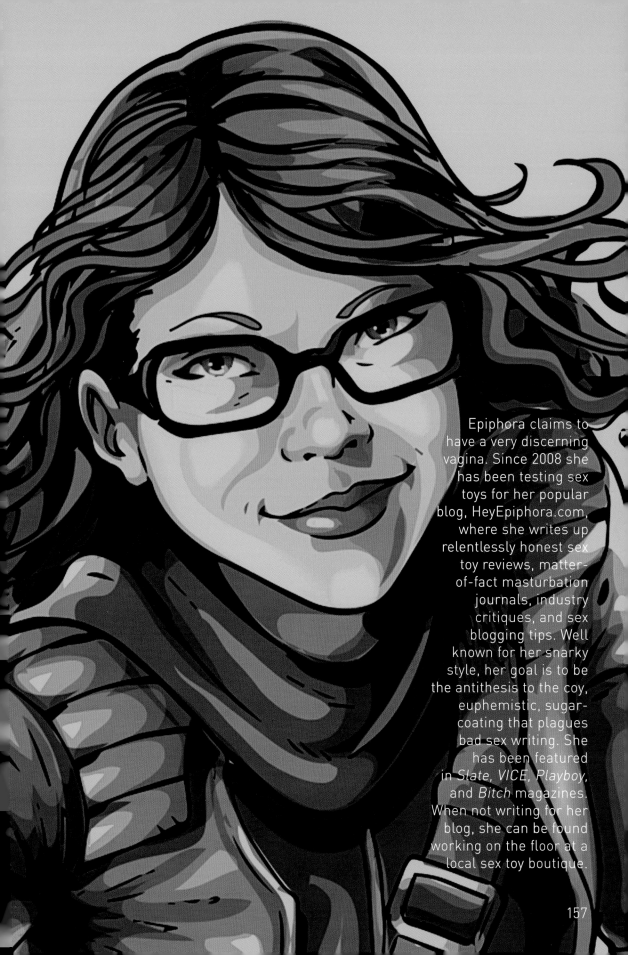

Epiphora claims to have a very discerning vagina. Since 2008 she has been testing sex toys for her popular blog, HeyEpiphora.com, where she writes up relentlessly honest sex toy reviews, matter-of-fact masturbation journals, industry critiques, and sex blogging tips. Well known for her snarky style, her goal is to be the antithesis to the coy, euphemistic, sugar-coating that plagues bad sex writing. She has been featured in *Slate*, *VICE*, *Playboy*, and *Bitch* magazines. When not writing for her blog, she can be found working on the floor at a local sex toy boutique.

LOVELIFE SHARE COUPLES RING BY OHMIBOD

2013
Body-safe silicone
ohmibod.com

Part of the Red Dot Design Award–winning Lovelife collection from OhMiBod, the Share vibrator is a heart-shaped ring featuring seven vibration patterns, one-button operation, and a USB-charging system. The splash-proof, 2.5"-long by 2.5"-wide silicone ring stretches to accommodate various sizes.

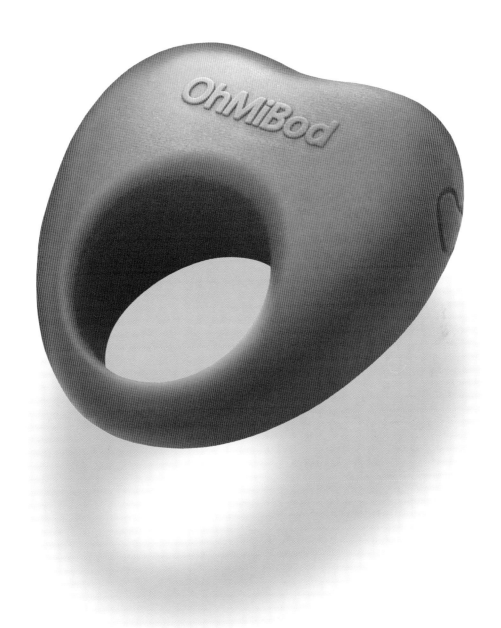

TOR 2
BY LELO
2012
Body-safe silicone
lelo.com

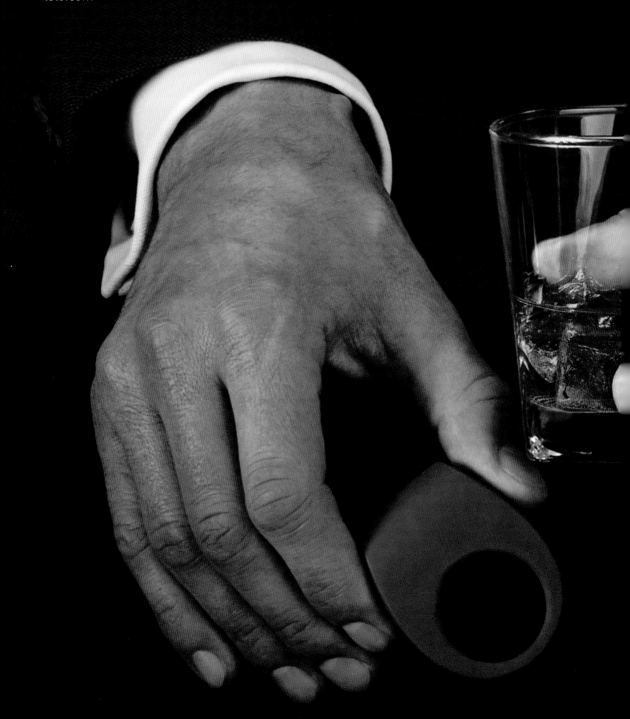

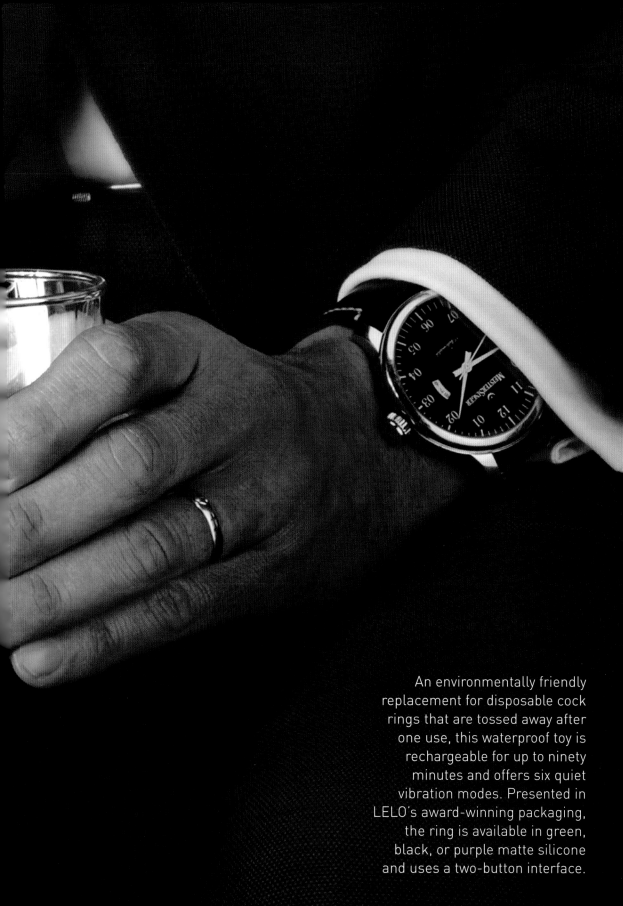

An environmentally friendly replacement for disposable cock rings that are tossed away after one use, this waterproof toy is rechargeable for up to ninety minutes and offers six quiet vibration modes. Presented in LELO's award-winning packaging, the ring is available in green, black, or purple matte silicone and uses a two-button interface.

TAILBUD
BY ROSEBUDS

1996

Horsehair, stainless steel, bronze

rosebuds.net

Part of a series of animal-tail themed butt plugs
from Rosebuds, Tailbud is made of a sweeping
mane of genuine horsehair. While the standard
version of the stainless-steel and bronze plug
measures 1.18" in diameter with a tail 15.8" long,
larger plug sizes and longer tails are also available.
In addition to black (shown), the horse tails come in
blond, auburn, grey, and flaxen hues. If you aren't
into horsing around, Rosebud offers many other
role-play-friendly plug styles, including synthetic
leopard, dog, or zebra tail designs.

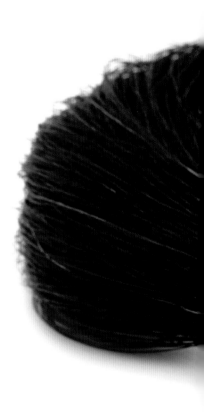

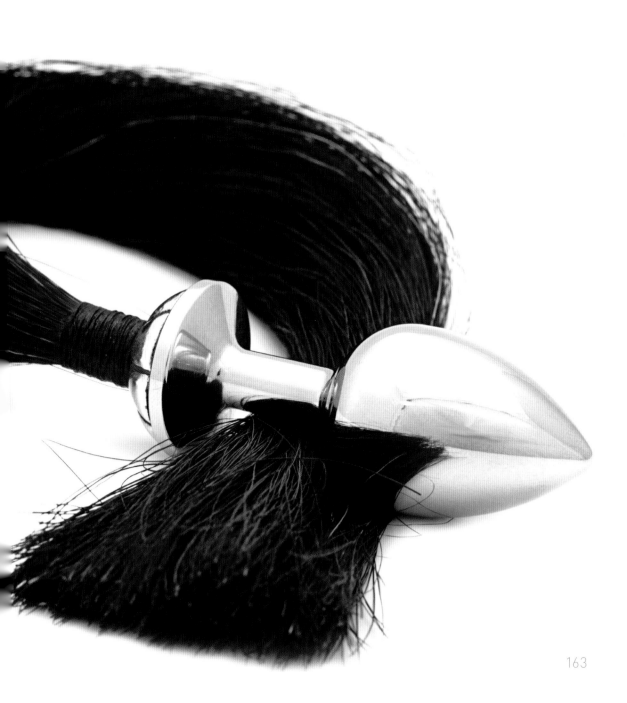

PINO
BY LELO

2014
Body-safe silicone, ABS plastic
lelo.com

Probably the *cockiest* of the cock
ring set, PINO was launched by
LELO in 2014 with great fanfare
as a toy designed exclusively for
bankers. Though it isn't made of
money, the stretchy, 100 percent
waterproof, rechargeable silicone
ring does come packaged in a box
with a pin-stripe shirt inlay, silver
cufflinks, and a matching money
clip engraved with the bankers'
mantra, *Always Be Closing*.

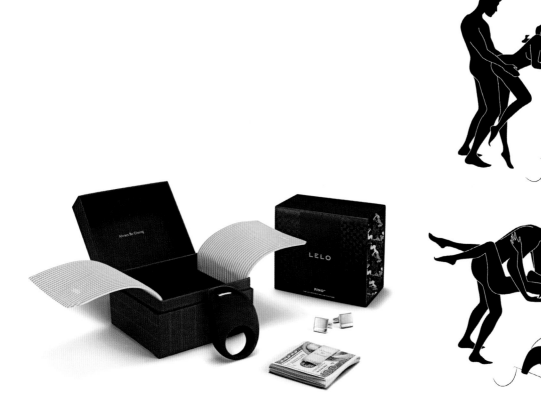

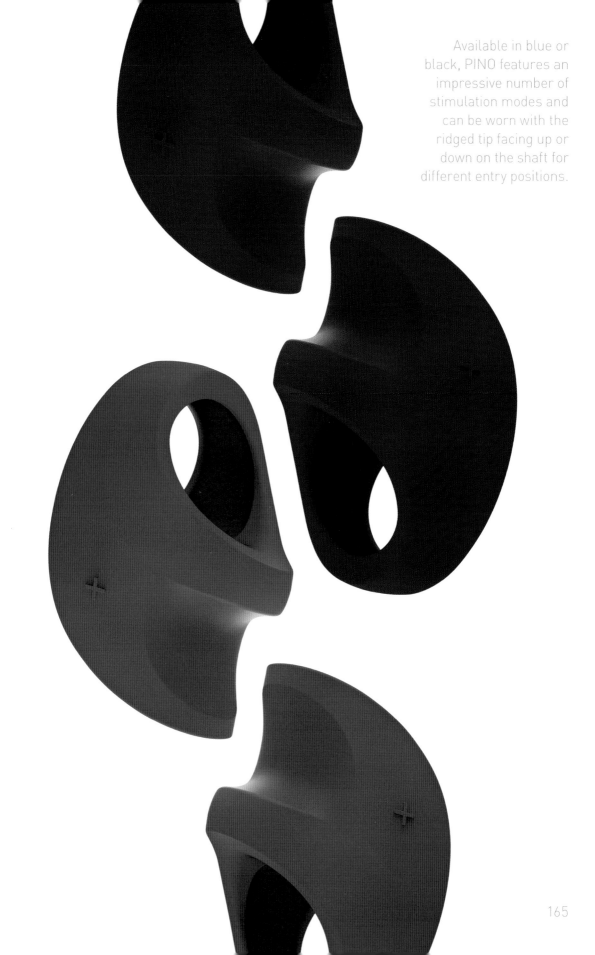

Available in blue or black, PINO features an impressive number of stimulation modes and can be worn with the ridged tip facing up or down on the shaft for different entry positions.

RINGO ERECTION RING
BY DEE LEE DOO

2014

Wood, water-thinned varnish

deeleedoo.com

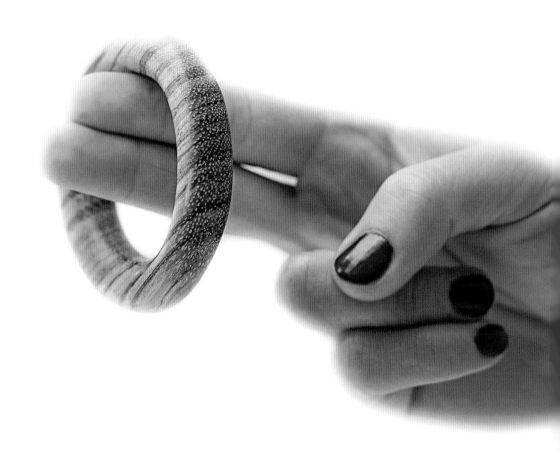

Handcrafted in Slovenia by
woodworker Iris Trstenjak, these
wooden cock rings join the artist's
growing collection of wooden dildos
and other personal accessories.
Designed to help men keep longer
erections, the waterproof rings are
handmade in three sizes out of one
of seven types of wood in the same
sanding and finishing process as
the dildo collection.

Q&A
METIS BLACK
FOUNDER AND PRESIDENT OF TANTUS INC.

Can you tell us a bit about how you helped bring silicone into the sex toy industry? What were the major challenges at the time?
Silicone sex toys were originally created by Gosnell Duncan, a disabled man, for himself and his friends. By 1997, when we began Tantus, there were less than ten manufacturers worldwide making silicone sex toys and production was limited to small boutiques. My goal with Tantus was to make mainstream silicone sex toys available to larger sex-toy-buying audiences. Here was the safest soft material for sex toys and yet almost no one knew about it or had access to it.

The first challenge was creating a process where production was efficient and scalable. That done, we started selling and making cold calls to bigger and bigger players in the business. We targeted trade shows to begin educating the distributors and the big chain stores. The first ANME (Adult Novelty Manufacturers Expo) Tantus attended was 2000. We were the first silicone toys there. Jelly toys were all the rage and when I'd mention that silicone could last a lifetime I lost the interest of many buyers—but they did like that it didn't smell. It took some perseverance but Tantus products were the first silicone toys in the Adam & Eve catalog. We made a lot of firsts.

Before silicone, what types of materials were sex toys made from?
Before silicone, the most common material for years had been rubber. PVC was actually relatively new when Tantus started making silicone toys. My guess is that both materials were made into sex toys about the same time—but the cost of PVC is so low and the method is so similar to rubber, that it was an immediate hit with the big manufacturers. Also as this was a business of "novelties," I think the mind-set was really geared to putting out toys at a twenty-dollar retail price point. It was hard for the major players to conceive of a higher-price-point toy without really evolved electronics.

How has your background working with artists helped your business?
I'm not really an artist, although Tantus had an artist originally as co-owner. Instead, I have a degree in humanities and I've marketed artists. Artists typically have difficulties selling themselves—you have to put your work up for critique, which is really hard. Because of my background though, I knew how to spin the perceived negatives, like that silicone could last a lifetime, in a way that brought about a different idea into the sales arena. If a dildo worked for a woman she wouldn't just buy one, just like she didn't just own one pair of black shoes in her closet.

Do you know who your typical customer is?
Tantus is the brand you buy when you know what you're buying. We are an educated sell but we also have been doing consumer and industry education for fifteen years now. Savvy is how I'd describe my customers, and they come in all shapes, sizes, nationalities, gender identities, and sexualities.

Do you design the toys yourself? How did you first get involved designing toys?
I do design a lot of toys, mainly on paper. I generally give the specifications for the toy and the general dimensions and let someone refine it either in sculpture or in a computer program. We make a prototype, review it, use it, and make sure it meets our expectations before bringing it to market. I mainly started making toys because at the time, there weren't toys I wanted to play with.

What other brands do you admire for their design-first approach to toy design?
I love Greg DeLong's Njoy toys, J. Snelling's creations on Rosebuds.net, and my all-time favorite designer is Ray Cirino. His old Inner Space toys are still some of my favorites to use and he was so ahead of his time with regards to healthy materials.

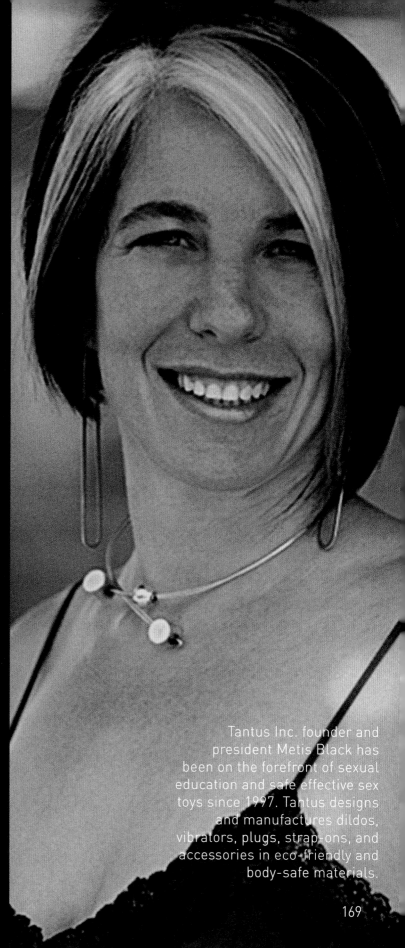

Any advice for a young sex toy designer? Advice for a first-time sex toy consumer?
Play with as many toys as you can before you make the jump to designer. Figure out what you love and don't follow the trends. I think so much comes to market that's never been played with and even those that have been tested, I wonder who their testers were. I know I had to do so much testing personally at first because my volunteer testers would just tell me "yes, it worked," which of course wasn't helpful at all.

What is your most popular toy?
Our most popular toy these days is hands-down our Super Soft C-Rings. I think men's toys are really just starting to make an impact in the industry, and we are all rethinking what a man's toy can be.

Tantus Inc. founder and president Metis Black has been on the forefront of sexual education and safe effective sex toys since 1997. Tantus designs and manufactures dildos, vibrators, plugs, strap-ons, and accessories in eco-friendly and body-safe materials.

PERFECT PLUG
BY TANTUS

2014
Body-safe silicone
tantusinc.com

For those interested in exploring anal play for the first time, it's imperative to start with the right toy—something small, easy to insert, and designed to help you do the job right. Only a finger's width in diameter, the Perfect Plug from Tantus has a velvety silicone surface with a narrow head for easy rear entry. The long, slender neck is insertable up to 3.5" and is tailored to be easily retainable (an anchor-shaped base tapers to fit between the cheeks). The plug also comes in a more advanced version (longer and wider) with an insertable bullet with three vibration speeds for more intense stimulation. Both options are boilable, bleachable, and dishwasher-safe, but not harness-compatible.

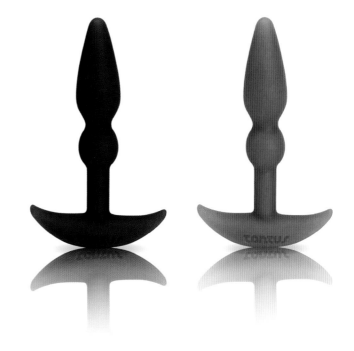

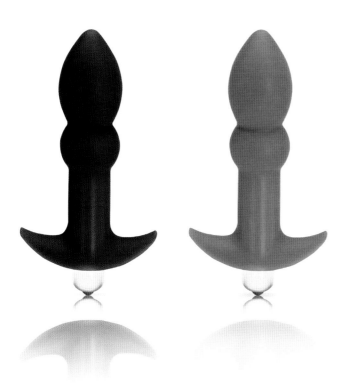

JBOA
BY VELV'OR

2012
Silicone, stainless steel
velv-or.com

Jelle Plantenga founded the Dutch brand Velv'or in 2006 after a search for a stylish cock ring left him high and dry. Working with several silversmiths, Plantenga developed the JCobra, a wishbone-shaped ring handcrafted in precious metal. While these ultra-luxe rings cost anywhere in the range from 1,600 to 90,000 euros depending on the material, Velv'or also offers a much more affordable Ready to Wear collection as well. Included in this group is the JBoa, a stylish lasso cock ring made of high-quality silicone string and a hand-finished stainless steel cylinder that is worn on the base of the penis close to the body. Once securely in place, JBoa can be enjoyed during sex or foreplay for up to thirty minutes.

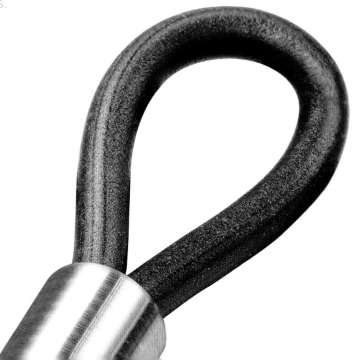

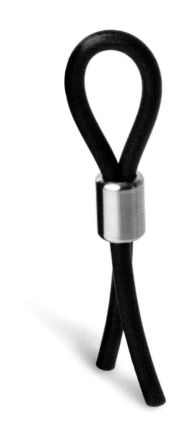

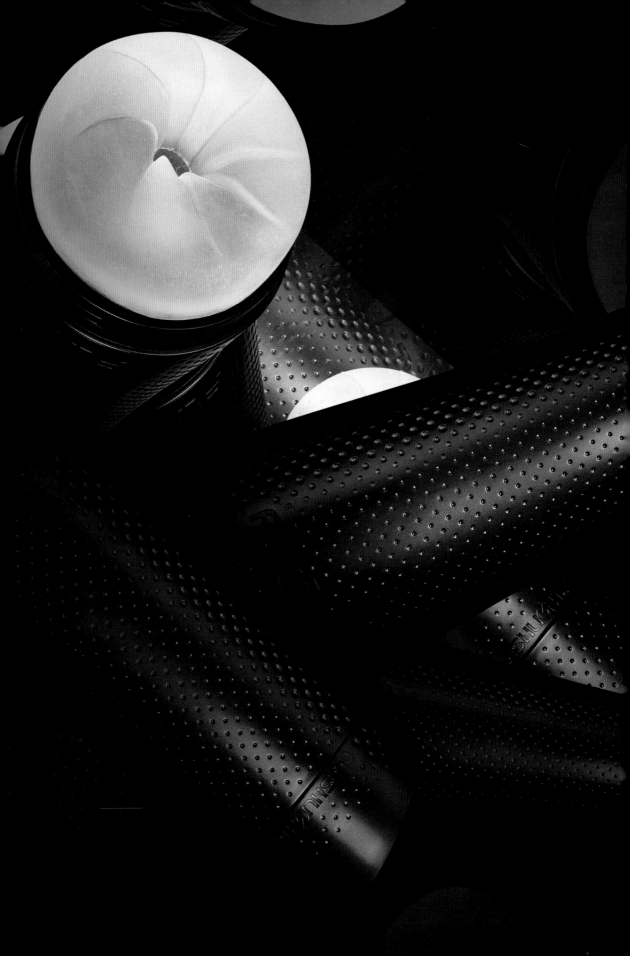

MALE STROKERS

PULSE II SOLO & DUO
BY HOT OCTOPUSS

2013
ABS plastic, body-safe silicone
hotoctopuss.com

According to Hot Octopuss, Pulse II is the world's first "Guybrator", a new type of device that applies state-of-the-art oscillating technology for male stimulation. Since a man does not have to have an erection to use it, Pulse II has also been touted by some as a revolutionary adult sexual health device. While the company makes no medical claims, they have received reports back from older customers, people with erectile dysfunction, and those suffering from mobility issues, that the toy has helped improve their sex lives.

Designed by Curventa Design Works, Pulse II comes in two versions: a Solo version created exclusively for male solo play, and Duo, designed for couples. To use, the man inserts his penis (flaccid or erect) into Pulse, making sure the frenulum is pressed against the toy's *PulsePlate*. As the sensation causes him to grow, the wings expand until the toy fits snugly around him.

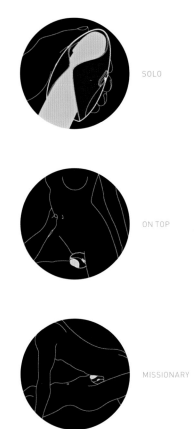

SOLO

ON TOP

MISSIONARY

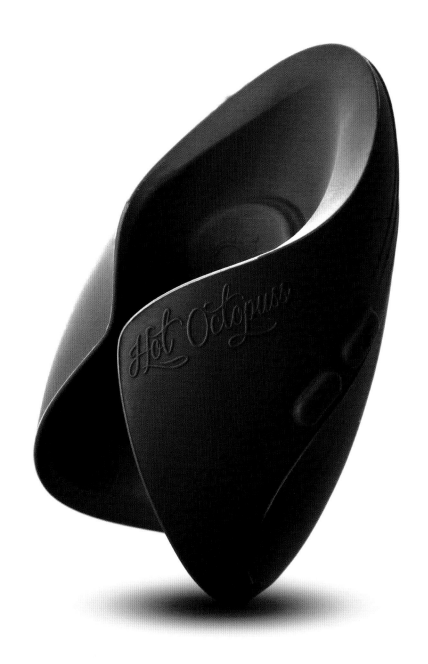

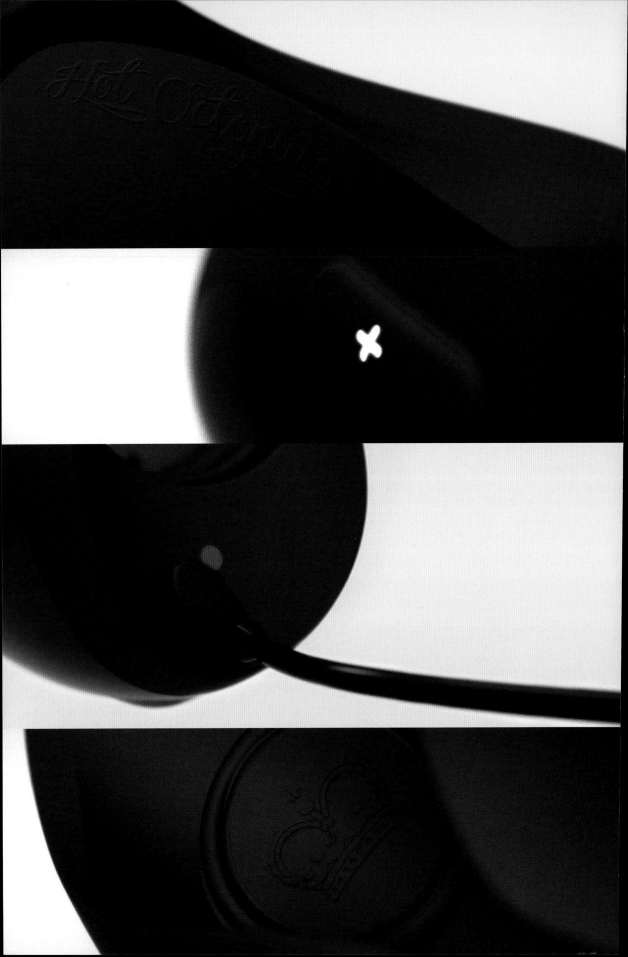

Pulse can be used either with lube as a masturbator or lubricant-free as a static stimulator. While the male experience will be the same with both toys, Duo offers a remote-controlled, vibrating underside of soft silicone for female partners. Both toys are rechargeable, 100 percent waterproof, and offer five pre-set vibration modes with adjustable intensities for the man.

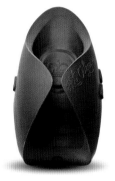

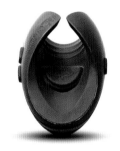

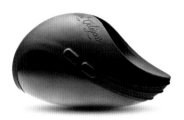

FLIP HOLE
BY TENGA

2008 – 2011
Thermoplastic elastomer (internal sleeve);
polycarbonate (case and slide cap)
tenga-global.com

While the main purpose of
the Flip Hole's hinged design
is to allow the toy to be more
easily cleaned and dried, it
also offers another benefit—
it lets users appreciate the
complex molding technology
inside. Each of the four
different versions (black,
shown), contains unique 3D
internal structures designed
to provide different sensations
during masturbation.
Depending on the style, Flip
Hole offers various levels
of solidity (strength of the
internal material), stimulation
(from light to strong), side
stimulation (tightness and
stimulation focused on the
sides), smoothness during
use, and suction gained from
pressing the center pad on
the device.

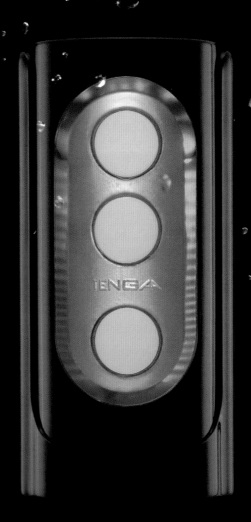

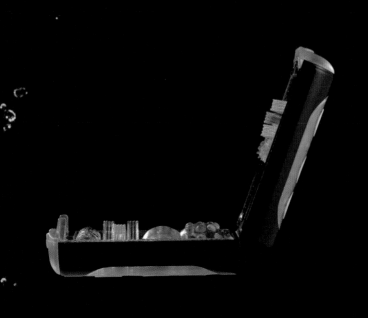

To use, users simply pull the holder from the body and apply lubricant. The Flip Hole is then reinserted into the holder and is ready for use. To clean, simply remove the toy from the holder, rinse with hand soap and water, and then rest on the holder until dry. Tenga claims that it can be reused up to fifty times with normal use, so be aware that it does have a shelf life.

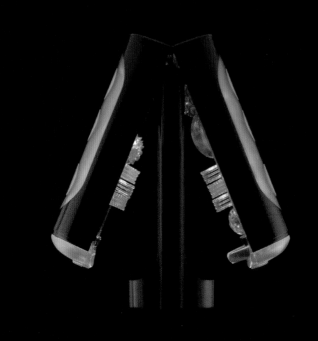

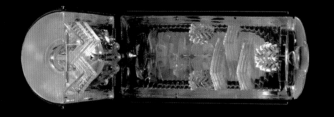

Q&A
JOELLEN NOTTE
SEX BLOGGER

redheadbedhead.com

How did you get started reviewing sex toys?
I never intended to review toys. I didn't even know that was something people did—I was pretty clueless when I started out—but about six months after I started my site people started asking to send me things to review.

What was the first sex toy that you owned? Can you tell us about that experience?
The first toy I ever owned was a white plastic vibrator I bought when I was twenty-one. I got it from a now-defunct website called *Little Shop of Sex Toys* (its logo was a big plant with vines holding sex toys). It was pretty crappy and didn't do much for me but because just about everything I had read/heard had said things to the tune of "I bought a vibrator and BOOM—explosive, mind-blowing orgasms!!!" I figured there was something wrong with me. I didn't try toys again for a long time after that.

Which types of sex toys do you feel are the best designed? Why do you think that is?
I struggle with this question because when you talk "types" of toys, everything that is done really well by one company has been done horribly by another. Fun Factory made the Stronic line of pulsators that I think are some the most innovative toys of the past couple of years and lower-end companies made cheaper "thrusters" making it hard to say pulsators are where it's at.

I want to say that we have wands down and cite Vibratex for the Mystic Wand and the Original Magic Wand, but then just this year a line of high-end wands came out that disappointed a lot of people.

I'm enjoying watching the progression and improvement in toy design as companies listen to feedback. When the We-Vibe 4 came out I was impressed to see that the new design addressed so many of the issues people had with the We-Vibe 3.

Which type of sex toy has a way to go in the design dept?
Cunnilingus simulators. I've yet to encounter one that struck me as well-designed for the task at hand. Also, masturbation sleeves. When it comes to the body-safe materials movement penises often get forgotten (I usually say dicks get the shaft—pun intended) but, come on! Let's have more awesome, silicone masturbation sleeves!

What are some of your top sex toy recommendations?
Vibratex Mystic Wand, Fun Factory Stronic Eins and Drei, Jimmyjane FORM 4, Blue Venus Waterproof Vibe, Vixen Creations Vixskin Mustang, Pure Wand, Tenga Eggs.

What should people avoid when shopping for sex toys?
Avoid toxic toys! The sex toy industry is completely unregulated and many companies not only use harmful ingredients in their toys but also package them deceptively.

My advice? Stick to non-porous, body-safe materials like silicone, glass, stainless steel, ceramic, wood, or ABS plastic and buy your toys from reputable retailers. My site redheadbedhead.com is home to the Internet's most comprehensive listing of sex-positive retailers, all of whom have a commitment to body-safe products and many of whom have online shops as well as brick-and-mortar locations.

Do you have any advice for sex toy designers?
Listen to your customers, listen to reviewers. Worry less about having the coolest looking toy and more about making it feel awesome. If you are designing a toy to stimulate a certain body part, make sure you consult people who have that body part—there's nothing worse than being told that an entire team of clitoris-less designers agrees that a toy is great for clitoral stimulation and if that's not my experience I must be using it wrong. Also, don't cut corners on materials or motors.

A writer, educator, and adult retail consultant, JoEllen Notte created The Redhead Bedhead when she decided she wanted to talk about sex on the Internet. She's written for multiple outlets, including Good Vibrations, *Life on the Swingset, Kinkly.com,* and her award-winning blog, RedheadBedhead.com. She has also toured the country teaching and visiting North America's best adult retail institutions on the first-of-its-kind Superhero Sex Shop Tour. Notte lives in Portland, Oregon, where likes to spend her day "writing, plotting to change the face of adult retail, geeking out about sex, and tasting all the beer."

183

TENGA 3D
BY TENGA

2011
Antibacterial thermoplastic elastomer, ABS plastic
tenga-global.com

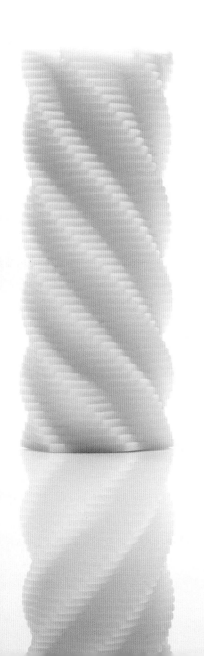

When it comes to penile masturbators (also known as strokers or sleeves), you can have the most realistic injection-molded vagina, mouth, or anus in the world on the receiving end, but everything that really matters happens on the inside of the toy. That's what puts the Red Dot Design Award-winning Tenga 3D in an entire class of its own.

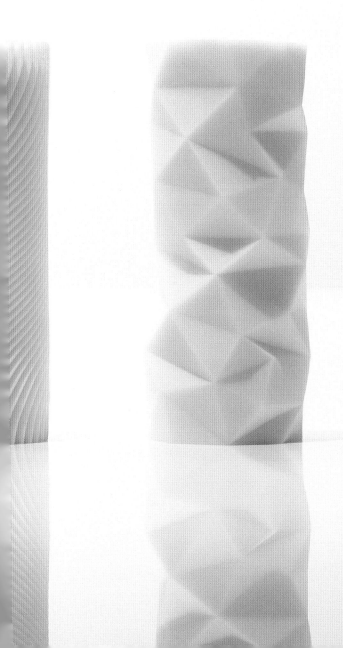
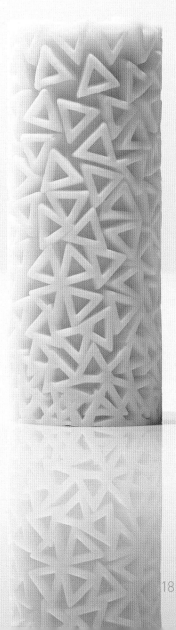

In order to use Tenga 3D, you must first turn the white, sculptural tube inside out. Each of the five textures, from spiral to polygonal, produces a different sensation. Pile, for example, uses stacked triangular protrusions that cascade from compact at the base to spread-out at the tip, while Module's randomly elevated blocks either rub or cling to the shaft to create the desired result. After use, simply wash out the antibacterial TPE tube and dry it in its case. This toy is beautiful and discreet enough to be left on display, so don't worry about hiding it in the back of the sock drawer.

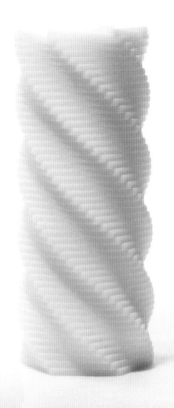

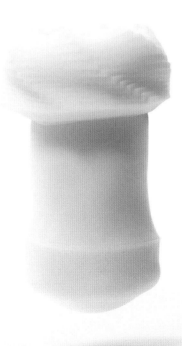

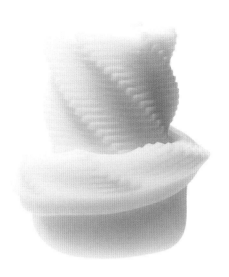

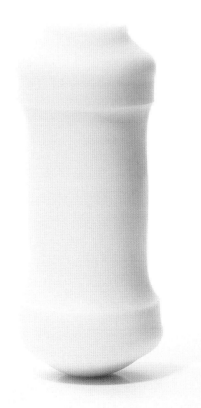

EGG LOVERS
BY TENGA

2011
Polypropylene (casing);
thermoplastic elastomer (sleeve)
tenga-global.com

Tenga introduced the first "Easy Beat" Egg, a pliable male pleasure sleeve, back in 2008. Thirteen different versions of the one-time-use disposable stroker are now available from the company, each with exterior packaging designs based on the patterns on the internal sleeves that create varied sensations for the user. Encased in a black and silvery-pink shell, the Egg Lovers design, shown here, features a heart-shaped pattern.

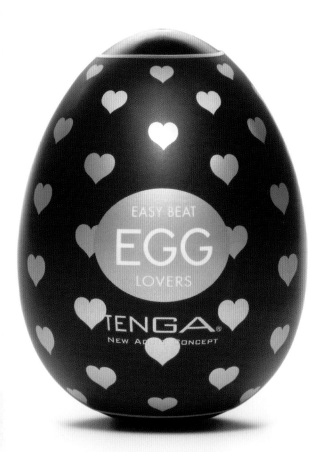
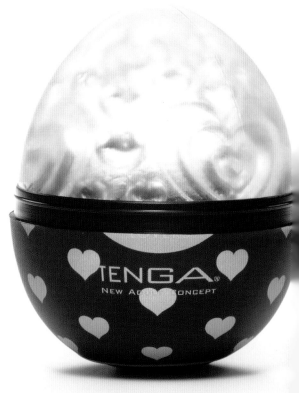

After first removing the shrink-wrapped packaging, users open the egg-shaped case, apply the lotion contained within the Egg into the sleeve, and then place it on the tip of the shaft. During use, the Egg's super-stretchy TPE material warms to body temperature and can cover almost any size penis.

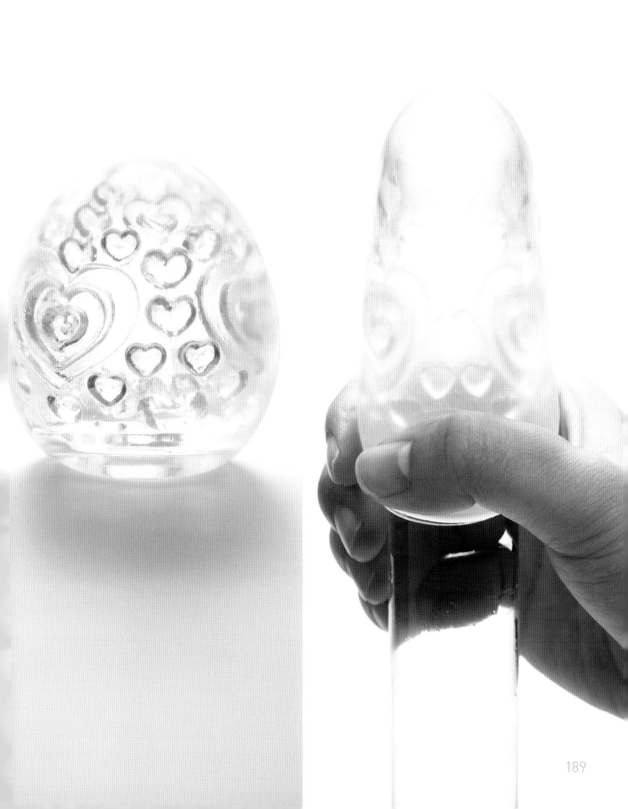

FLIGHT
BY FLESHLIGHT

2012
Mineral-based elastic thermo
polymer (sleeve), polypropylene
fleshlight.com

When not in use, traditional
Fleshlight strokers can
be hidden in plain sight
due to their discreet cases
that resemble flashlights.
The Flight Pilot and Flight
Instructor, with external
cases that could double
as fancy thermoses, are
intended to be easier to
store and take on the road.

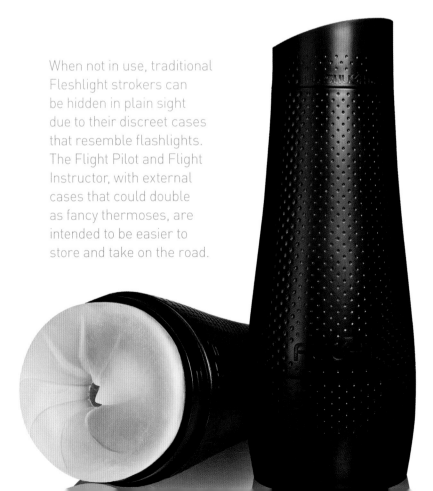

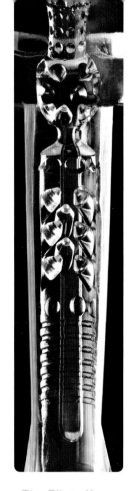

The Pilot offers a number of internal textures (bumps, fingers, and ribs) and canal-width changes, while Instructor offers a "less turbulent" or smoother experience. Both offer a total insertable length of 8" and come with an adapter that enables both shower-mounting and virtual reality play.

Q&A
SHAUNA MEI
FOUNDER & CEO OF AHALIFE.COM & AHANOIR.COM

Why did you decide to launch AHAnoir?
When we started AHAlife it was Chinese New Year. We have an email program with new discoveries, and I got approached by the founders of Jimmyjane to launch Jimmyjane on the site, and I thought it was amazing but didn't know if it was appropriate for me to send that out to my audience on AHAlife who are looking for luxury high-design items. It was the Year of the Rabbit and I wanted to send out one of Jimmyjane's top products, a mini-rabbit vibrator that was gorgeous. I sent out an email that said "welcome to the year of the rabbit" and it was the product we promoted that day. It just sold like crazy. So I started to look more into these types of products.

I started learning about the industry and found there really was nothing elegant out there that puts together highly curated and unique products that allow people to buy these things comfortably at home. So we launched a special section called The Back Room, and we started collecting really cool sex toys, lingerie, accessories, etc., and that whole segment of our site became a huge performer. That's when I came up with the idea to launch a sister site called AHAnoir so that I could really market specifically to people that would enjoy this kind of content and curation.

What product type do you think has the most room for growth?
I actually think we need more brands like William Wilde and Maison Close, not just lingerie but really more sexy outfits that people can wear if you are into that lifestyle. There are just not enough options out there and not enough designers to fit into that space.

Also, there are a lot of people that do these one-offs—but not real brands—that do these accessories like great leather whips and handcuffs and blindfolds, but not enough that are really high quality. There are a lot of brands that sell these things that are a notch lower than I would like to carry on my site. There is not a brand that is dominating the entire S&M accessory space with higher quality products, and with *Fifty Shades of Grey* that's become a topic of a lot of interest.

Do you have any favorite brands?
I think I have a soft spot for Jimmyjane because they are the reason I got into this whole world and I think that they continue to make really high-quality products that are well packaged.

I am not a guy, obviously, but I love the Alpha One. They are these male masturbators that look like mini-speakers, and I think they are gorgeous. The one I think is beautiful is called The Gold Ring and it is 24k gold-plated metal and comes with this unique silicone that feels really nice for solo play. It's $400, so it's a luxury product. We actually had a pop-up shop with Hotel Particulier, an amazing experimental art space here in New York, and this is one of the products that we curated and it got the most engagement.

I also think the Tenga eggs are such a fun concept, and it's a surprise. I love people that are pushing the envelope—these gorgeous high-end dildos that are done by Crystal Delights, they do the butt plugs with crystals and diamonds and they are all hand-blown glass sculptures. I think they are just really beautiful.

What are the most popular products on the site?
It might surprise you. On AhaNoir one of our top selling product is this anal butt plug that has a My Little Pony tail. I think it's just funny because it's such an odd, unique item and we added it originally because we thought it was cool but it's actually a top-seller.

Our lubricant section has done really well for us and some of our bodysuits, like William Wilde, have done well. Lingerie in general has been selling well for us, like pieces from the Something Wicked and Maison Close. We have this thing called sexual mask flavors, there are these like breath mint strips that you get to use prior to oral sex, and those things have been selling really well, which I think is interesting.

Love is Art is a kit we have that you can have sex on that does really well for us. It's a canvas and you have sex on it with your partner and it creates an abstract painting with paint.

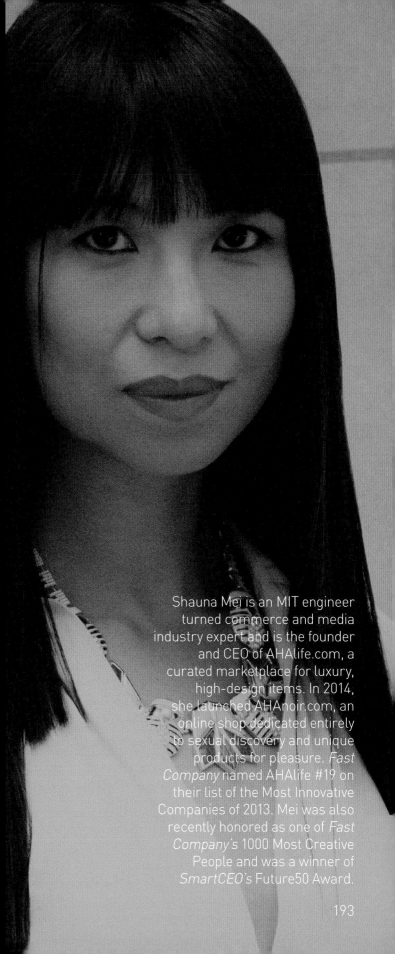

Has the stigma towards sex toys been improving?
I think having AHAnoir being associated with AHAlife is an advantage. Our mission statement is to help everyone live their life to the fullest and there is no reason why your sexual well-being shouldn't be part of that. We talk about it in a very holistic way and I think it really removes the stigma around the topic. Our customers are a lot more comfortable because they see AHAnoir is associated with a luxury site that they already know and trust, and there is not all this taboo associated with it.

What trends do you see in erotic product design?
I touched on this already, but male masturbators have really come out in the past couple of years and are really selling, which is pretty surprising to me actually, and another trend in general is higher-quality products. I think historically people didn't think of sex toys as being serious. They thought they were made of plastic in China, and now we see that people are spending substantial money. We actually have sold a solid gold dildo on our site that's thousands of dollars.

Do you know who is your typical customer?
We seeded it with a lot of our audience in New York City and since then we actually get orders from all over the United States. It's actually been pretty surprising. We have a very loyal, engaged New York audience that are members of AHAlife as well as friends and my personal network, so we seeded it with a little bit over two thousand people in New York and it's been really engaged with that core group. At AHAlife, we have more of an urban customer, while AHAnoir is urban and suburban all over the country. It's both men and women, about a fifty-fifty split.

Shauna Mei is an MIT engineer turned commerce and media industry expert and is the founder and CEO of AHAlife.com, a curated marketplace for luxury, high-design items. In 2014, she launched AHAnoir.com, an online shop dedicated entirely to sexual discovery and unique products for pleasure. *Fast Company* named AHAlife #19 on their list of the Most Innovative Companies of 2013. Mei was also recently honored as one of *Fast Company*'s 1000 Most Creative People and was a winner of *SmartCEO*'s Future50 Award.

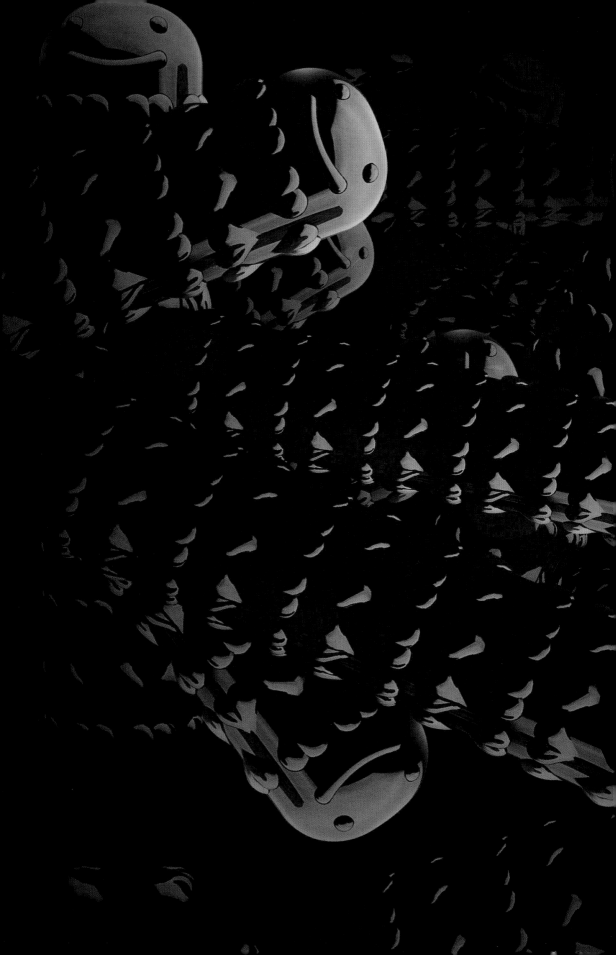

DILDOS & HARNESSES

DILDIY
BY CUNICODE

2013
3D-printed materials
cunicode.com/works/dildiy

In the foreseeable future, anyone
with a 3D printer at home will be
able to download some software
and custom design—among endless
other things—their very own sex
toys. In fact, the Barcelona-based
Cunicode, mainly run as a one-man
shop by Bernat Cuni, has already
developed a concept app that will
allow customers to shape and design
a custom, 3D-printed sex toy.

According to Cuni, a product
designer specializing in digital
fabrication, the project was initiated
in a workshop held by the online 3D
printing service i.materialise and
the UK-based software company
Digital Forming, where his firm
tested a new generation of tools
that allow personalization and mass
customization through 3D printing.

Cunicode is also working on
a generative design approach (where
the output is generated by a set of
rules or an algorithm), incorporating
personal inputs such as sound to
define the toy's volume and details.
While the project is still in the
prototype stage, Cuni envisions the
toys will be printed in food-safe
ceramics, giving them a luxurious
look and feel.

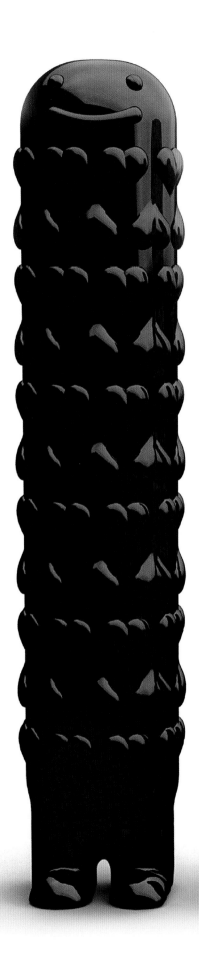

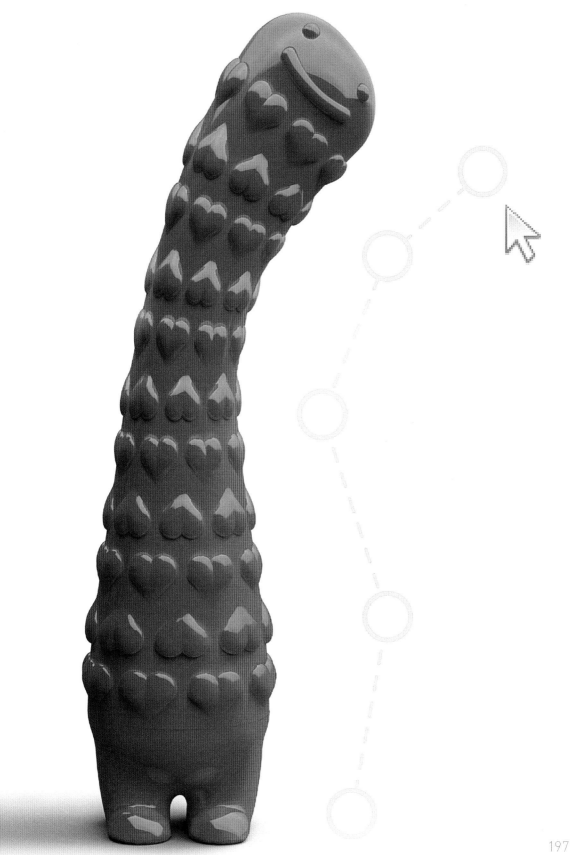

197

Q&A
IRIS TRSTENJAK
DIRECTOR, DEE LEE DOO

How did you first get involved designing wooden dildos?
It just happened in the workshop. While creating different kinds of things, this was one of my ideas, and all I had to do is to make one. It looked very beautiful. Of course, I also tried it out, and it was very pleasant. Then I made some more.

What has been the biggest challenge in the design process?
Well, the biggest challenge was testing all the shapes we made and also getting more opinions so that we could decide which shapes are the most practical, satisfying, and convenient for use. Thanks to all my friends, we managed to test them all and get an honest critique.

Which types are wood are most popular with your customers?
It is very different, with no rules. Different types of people have many different wishes for the choice of the wood type and the model of the dildo. The dildos we chose fit most personalities. The wood types are very different, so I think that there is something for everyone.

Any advice for other young women interested in designing objects for sex play?
My story has thankfully, and surprisingly, attracted a lot of people. All of the responses were very positive. I am just getting into the industry, but have to say that there are a lot of people prepared to help, give advice, and show the way. The recipe is that you just have to work, make your own stuff, and most importantly, have the guts to show it to people. Make it good, stand behind it, and tell your story.

Has there been any issue with convincing people that wooden toys are safe to use?
Not really. The wood is worked with a lot of care and precision, smoothed to perfection, and coated with a safe, certified finish. Our dildos are made in beautiful shapes. Everybody knows the best one for him/herself. The most important thing is that the user must be comfortable with the product in every way. Mine, which I store in a glass cabinet, satisfies me just by staring at it.

What are you working on next?
We are developing the dildos and making them more than just dildos. Soon we will put some of our new products on the market, so we are always working and making new things.

When not waitressing, the Slovenia-based designer Iris Trstenjak works at Dee Lee Doo, her woodshop where she produces handmade, all-natural wooden dildos and other accessories. Trstenjak, who has studied multimedia and wood technology, hopes that one day Dee Lee Doo will become a recognizable brand for all-natural erotic accessories.

HANDCRAFTED WOODEN DILDOS BY DEE LEE DOO

2013
Wood, water-thinned varnish
deeleedoo.com

Handcrafted in Slovenia by woodworker Iris Trstenjak, these all-natural dildos bring an entirely new meaning to the term *woodie*. Made from one of seven different wood options—from maple to wenge the pieces come in a range of sizes and shapes for different uses and sensations. No need to worry about splinters—the dildos require multiple stages of careful sanding and are then finished with several layers of environmentally friendly, water-thinned transparent varnish to make them waterproof.

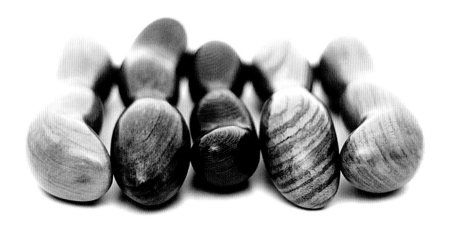

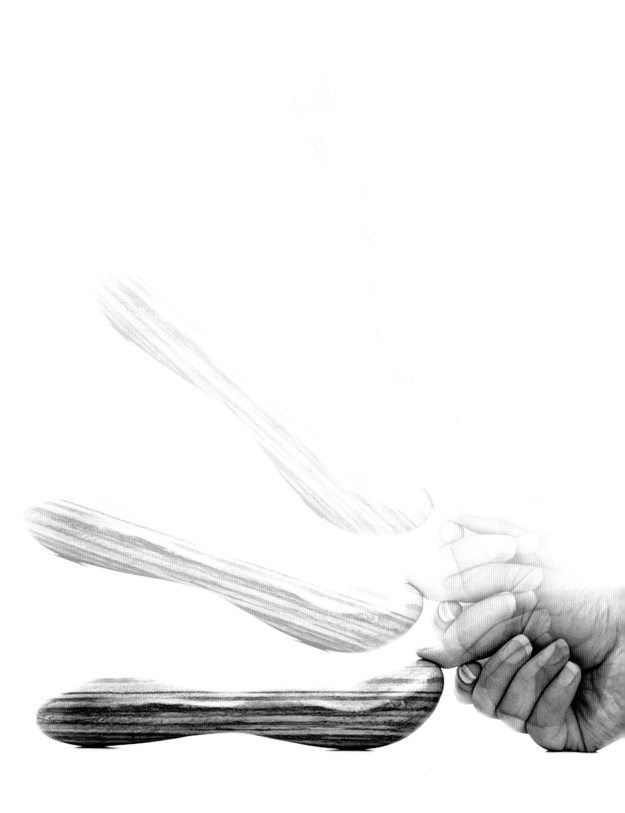

ALOE
BY DISCOH

2008
Medical-grade silicone
discoh.com

Designed by the Valenica, Spain-
based design firm Discoh,
Aloe is an elongated, leaf-like
dildo made of flexible medical
silicone that will appeal to those
who want to simulate a more
"natural" experience in the
bedroom. According to Discoh,
Aloe was created as a decorative
object that only reveals its true
purpose once it's unpacked.
The package design, therefore,
was as important as the design
of the object itself, and the firm
found inspiration in typical gifts
exchanged between couples,
such as plants, flowers, and
perfume bottles.

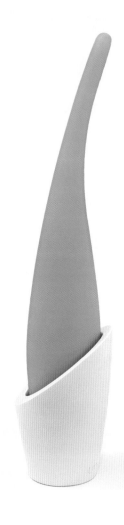

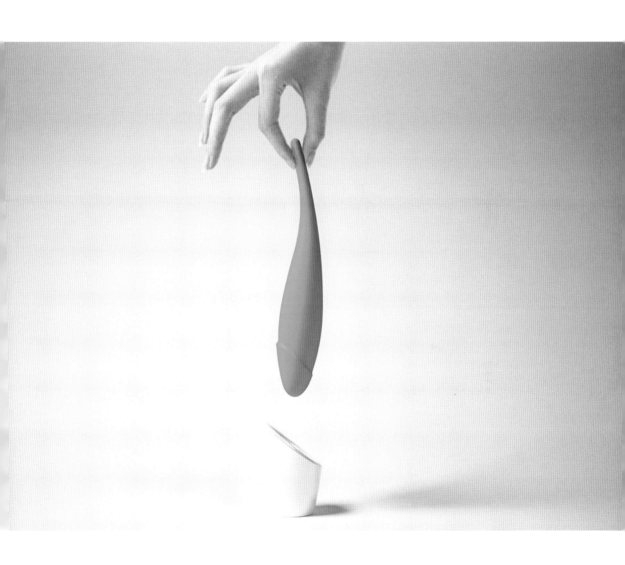

BLUE LEATHER TASSEL STRAP & CERAMIC DILDO BY SHIRI ZINN

2009
Napa lambskin,
ceramic, gold leaf
shirizinn.com

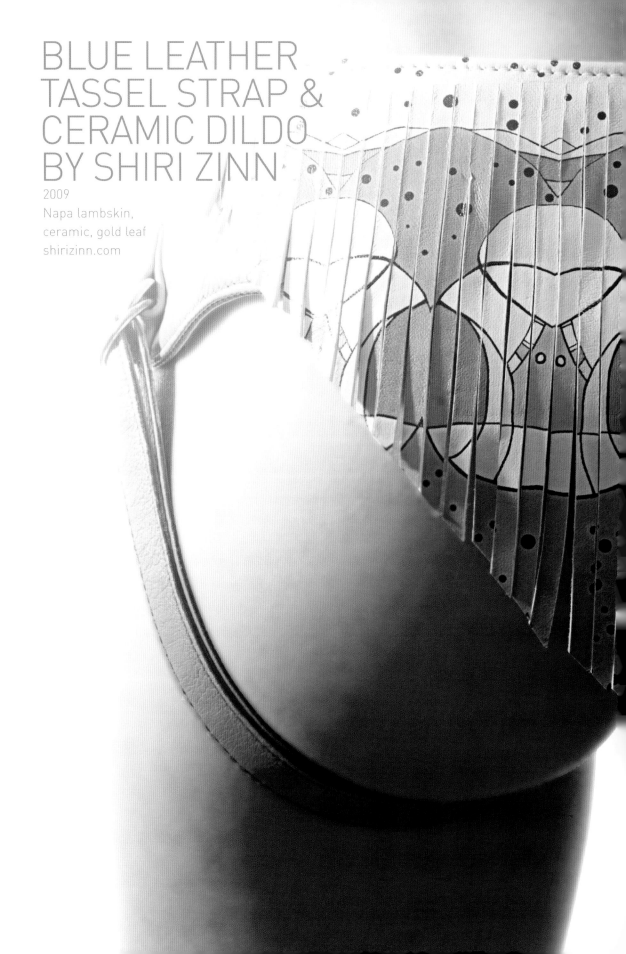

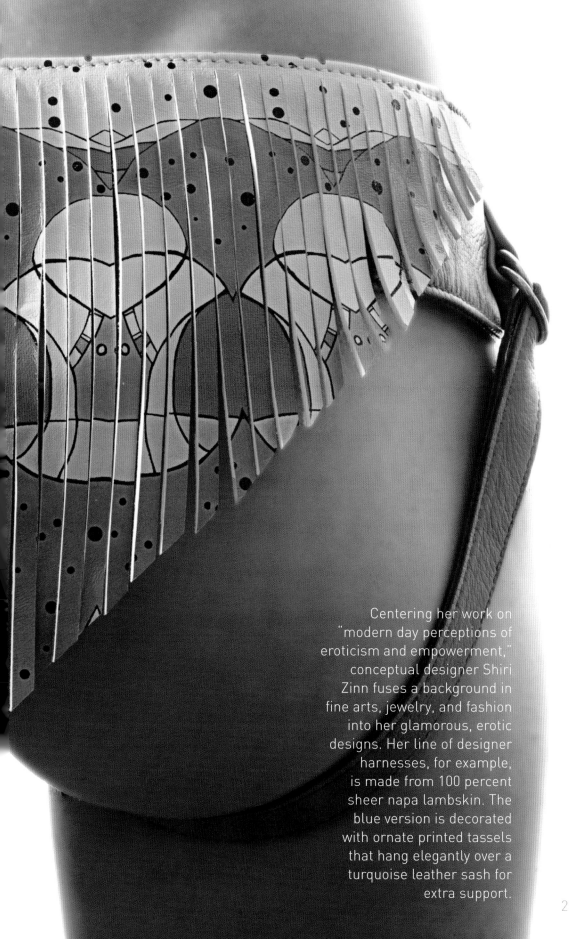

Centering her work on "modern day perceptions of eroticism and empowerment," conceptual designer Shiri Zinn fuses a background in fine arts, jewelry, and fashion into her glamorous, erotic designs. Her line of designer harnesses, for example, is made from 100 percent sheer napa lambskin. The blue version is decorated with ornate printed tassels that hang elegantly over a turquoise leather sash for extra support.

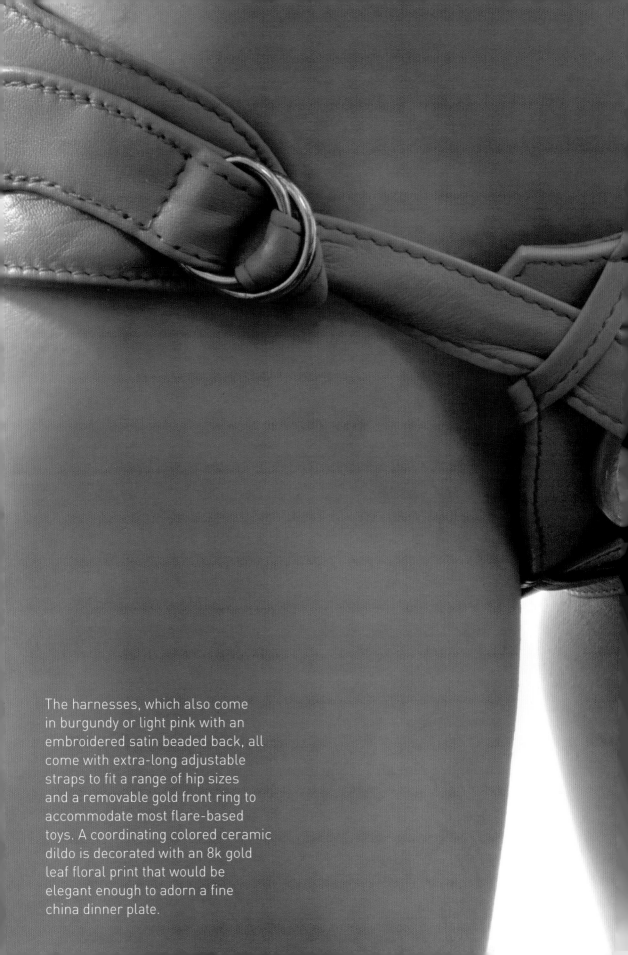

The harnesses, which also come in burgundy or light pink with an embroidered satin beaded back, all come with extra-long adjustable straps to fit a range of hip sizes and a removable gold front ring to accommodate most flare-based toys. A coordinating colored ceramic dildo is decorated with an 8k gold leaf floral print that would be elegant enough to adorn a fine china dinner plate.

Q&A
KARIM RASHID
INDUSTRIAL DESIGNER
& INTERIOR ARCHITECT

In 2012, you designed a dildo called Mr. Pink for Fun Factory. How did you get involved with that project? Was this your first sex toy collaboration?
I previously designed some vibrators for Mila in London and created the Karimsutra, which is landscape living furniture that helps create thirty-six sexual positions. The Karimsutra was a one-off for the Museum of Sex in New York City. I originally worked with Fun Factory by designing their flagship store in Berlin and now we've added another store in Munich. They asked me to design some sex toys. What I proposed were toys that were more "design" than what they were looking for, but they saw a freehand sketch I had done and liked it and thought it could translate well into a dildo. The interesting part of it is the technology where a floro pink inner core is molded firstly and then a send-over mold is produced giving it an ethereal, evocative feeling.

Were you presented with a design brief or given free reign?
Fun Factory gave me free reign with Mr. Pink. I wanted to create a playful toy for a multitude of sexual behaviors and a blurring of our needs and desires. Mr. Pink is a functional object but also full of desire, emotion, and passion. The fine line for me was to do something tasteful, not too literal, and a bit abstract.

How long was the design process? Was the comfort-level equal to other projects or did the team find a sex toy more challenging?
It is no different from any other project. Once marginal and taboo, sex and sex toys, like design, are now ubiquitous. The underlying narratives of sex toys, like perfume bottles for example, are desire, form, seduction, beauty, and physicality. Design is a public subject. Design is now shaping every aspect of living so the final frontier is to shape a better sex life.

Have you worked on any other objects for erotic pleasure since the collection?
Yes, I am working on a limited-edition sex chair inspired from the idea of creating landscapes for relaxation and a multitude of behaviors, as well as a new vibrator for Fun Factory.

Any particular product type you'd like to tackle?
I would love to continue the exploration of sex and furniture and how it can create a more dynamic experience.

What advice would you give designers looking to improve the design of the dildo?
I honestly believe that there is little to improve. There are some perfectly high-performing toys in the market (and many variations). I think that the only real improvement is in the technology.

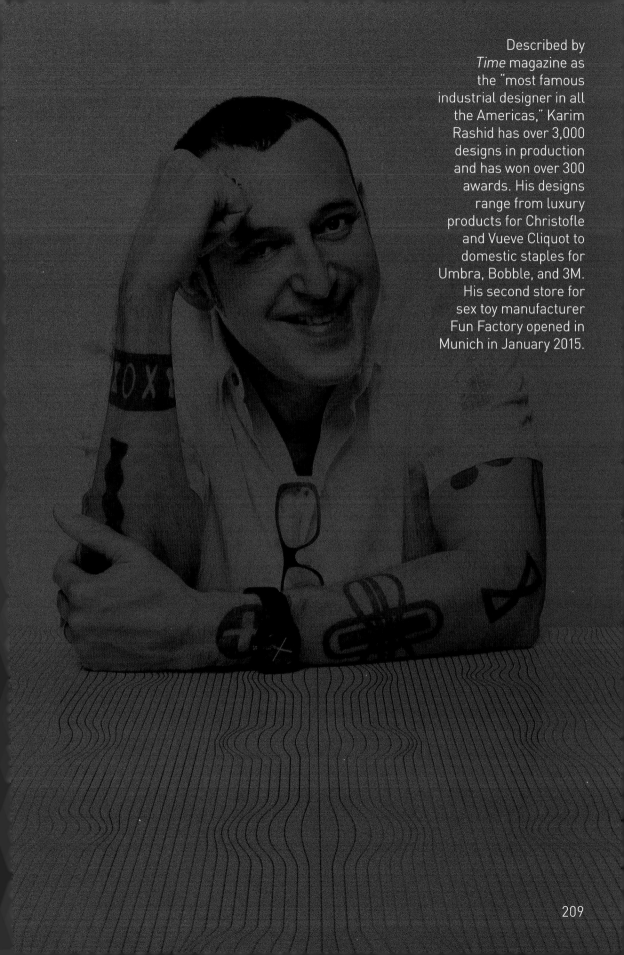

Described by *Time* magazine as the "most famous industrial designer in all the Americas," Karim Rashid has over 3,000 designs in production and has won over 300 awards. His designs range from luxury products for Christofle and Vueve Cliquot to domestic staples for Umbra, Bobble, and 3M. His second store for sex toy manufacturer Fun Factory opened in Munich in January 2015.

MR. PINK
DESIGNED BY KARIM RASHID
FOR FUN FACTORY

2012
Medical-grade silicone
funfactory.com

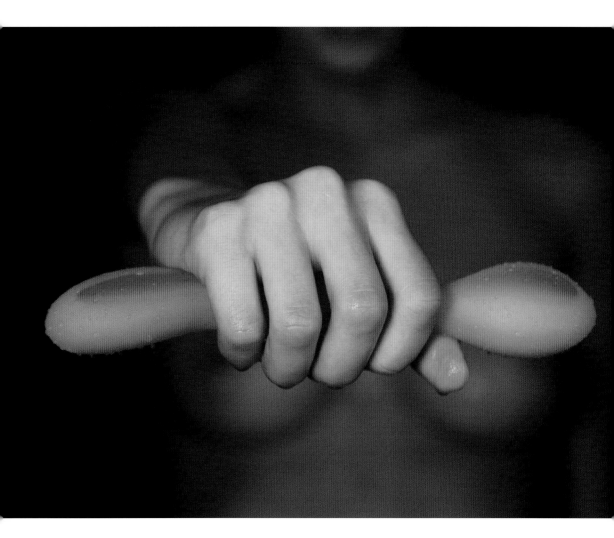

Those familiar with the work of world-renowned industrial designer Karim Rashid won't be surprised by the choice of Rashid's signature pink for his designer dildo for Fun Factory. Designed for vaginal use, Mr. Pink features a pink core surrounded by transparent silicone that has been poured and formed by hand in Germany. The 7.8"-long, waterproof toy has a velvety soft surface and can be used from either end. Rashid first worked with Fun Factory on the design of their flagship store in Berlin, and more recently, on a Munich store for the company.

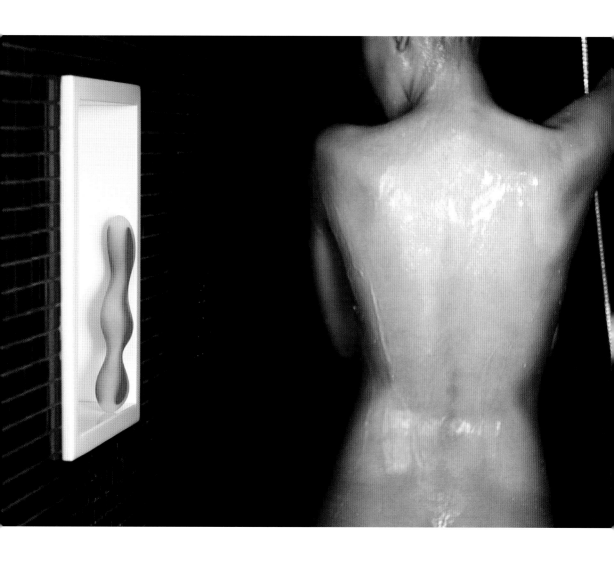

HIGH PRIESTESS BELT & BANANA SUNDAE DILDO BY WONDERPUSS OCTOPUS

2010

Silicone, latex, dimensional fabric paint

wonderpussoctopusink.com

Wonderpuss Octopus, a.k.a. the Brooklyn-based artist PJ Linden, explores "texture fetishism" with her incredibly detailed, multilayered strata of 3D fabric paint, acrylic, and latex (see page 138 for more info). The High Priestess Belt is a functional harness that was displayed at the Museum of Sex in New York City. The belt is shown here with the Banana Sundae Dildo, a chocolate sauce- and candy sprinkle-covered confectionery created out of 3D fabric paint. Intended as a piece of sculpture, the dildo is not recommended for internal use.

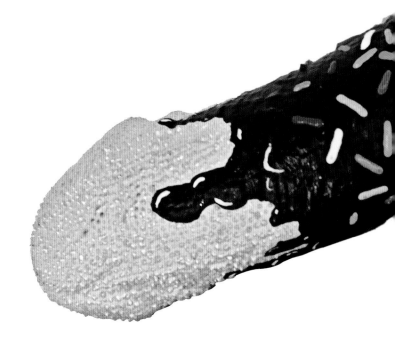

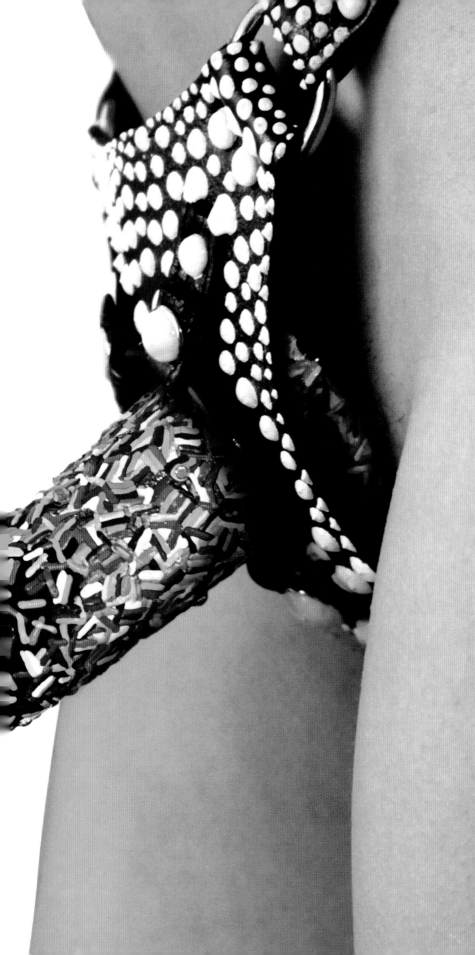

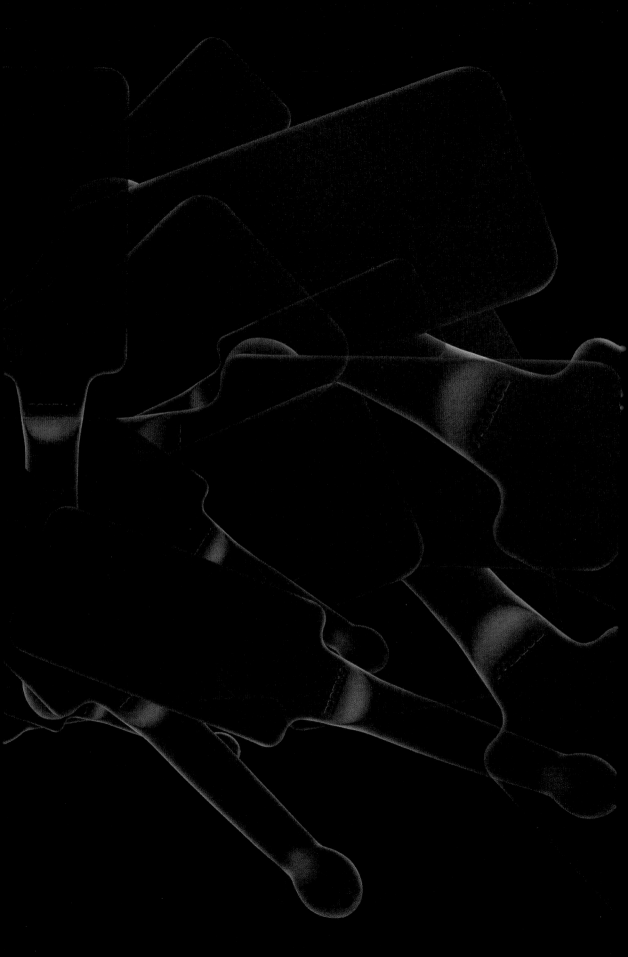

LIGHT BDSM

SONORAN WHIP
BY DEE LEE DOO

2013
Wood, water-thinned varnish, leather
deeleedoo.com

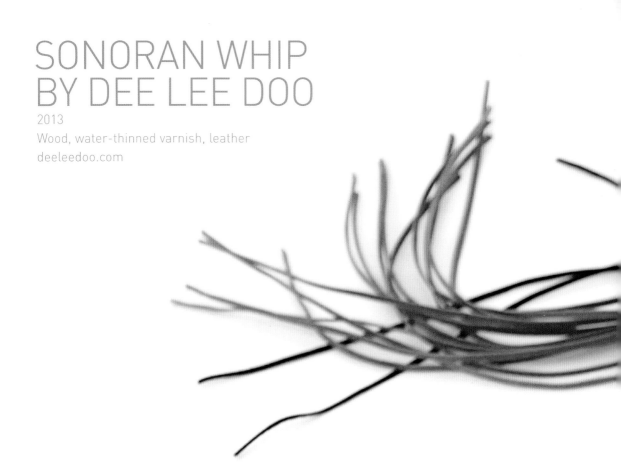

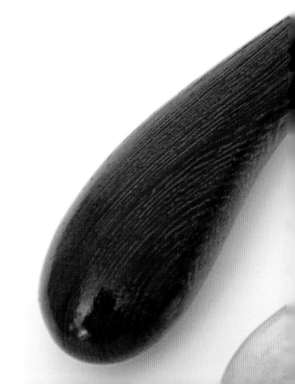

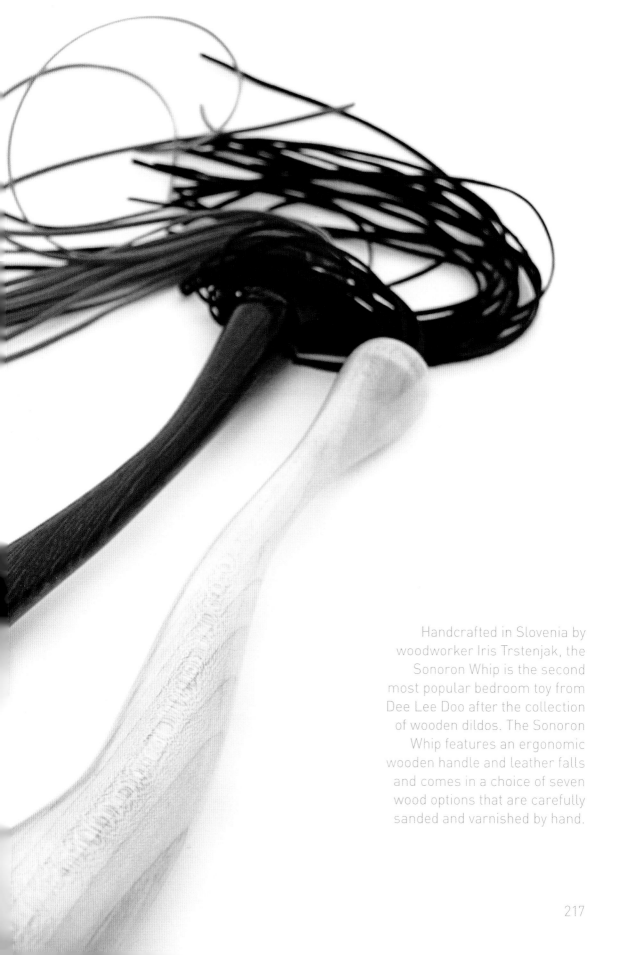

Handcrafted in Slovenia by woodworker Iris Trstenjak, the Sonoron Whip is the second most popular bedroom toy from Dee Lee Doo after the collection of wooden dildos. The Sonoron Whip features an ergonomic wooden handle and leather falls and comes in a choice of seven wood options that are carefully sanded and varnished by hand.

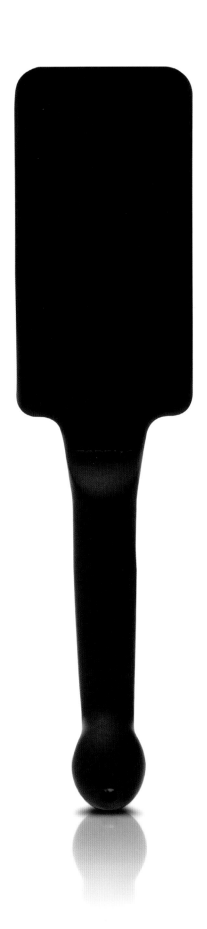

PLUNGE PADDLE
BY TANTUS

2013
Body-safe silicone
tantusinc.com

This flexible paddle for the "advanced enthusiast" comes with a bulbous head and smooth shaft that is insertable up to 6", doubling its potential for play in the bedroom. Boilable, bleachable, and dishwasher-safe, the hypoallergenic paddle is made from Tantus's own formula of 100 percent ultra-premium silicone.

Q&A
MONA DARLING
DOMINATRIX &
MOMMY BLOGGER
darlingpropaganda.com

Was it always your intention to review sex toys on the blog?
I wasn't going to, but the allure of free sex toys was just too great. I try to review something about once a month. Occasionally I will have companies send my readers something to review, which has worked out well as they get a free toy and the rest of my readers get a fresh perspective.

Favorite sex toys for the dungeon? Favorite toys for home?
My favorite sex toys for my home and for my dungeon differ quite a bit. For my home, my We-Vibe is a favorite, as is my Share [double-ended dildo by Fun Factory]. Those are way too intimate for use in the dungeon. I'm also a huge fan of the simple Wahl 7 Way vibrator. For the dungeon I enjoy canes, dragon tails, and other impact toys. Recently, Tantus sent me a silicone paddle with an ergonomic and insertable handle called The Plunge, which has become a favorite.

Do you think that the stigma towards sex toys has changed in the past few years?
I think it most definitely has! When I was in college, sex toys were nearly impossible to buy. When you did find them, they were made of unsafe materials or marketed as a back massager.

Now every large city and even many small cities have a clean, well-lighted place to buy toys. Even if you don't have one in your town, the Internet has a plethora of places to buy them. Even Amazon sells them. As someone who has been in the sex industry for over twenty years, I have watched as the Internet has made all things sexual easier to get, and therefore easier to talk about.

Do you think there is a particular person or company that is doing a good job helping to break down the stigma related to sex toys?
I don't think any conversation about breaking down stigma around sex toys can be had without acknowledging Good Vibrations in San Francisco for being the first clean, well-lighted place for sex toys, as well as Carol Queen for tirelessly promoting the benefits of masturbation. It's a rough job, but someone has to do it! I think there are always new amazing sex educators coming onto the scene, some of the most notable would be Ducky Doolittle and Tristan Taormino. I would also want to acknowledge women like Courtney Trouble and April Flores (plus-size pornography stars) for teaching people that skinny doesn't equal sexy.

What are your favorite blogs/sites that review sex toys?
I love Epiphora (heyepiphora.com) and Erika Moen of Oh Joy Sex Toy (ohjoysextoy.com). Epiphora is snarky and real. Erika Moen does a great comic strip using each product. Both of them are entertaining as well as educational. Both offer their opinion, good or bad, and I feel like I can trust them. Also, neither uses cutesy euphemisms.

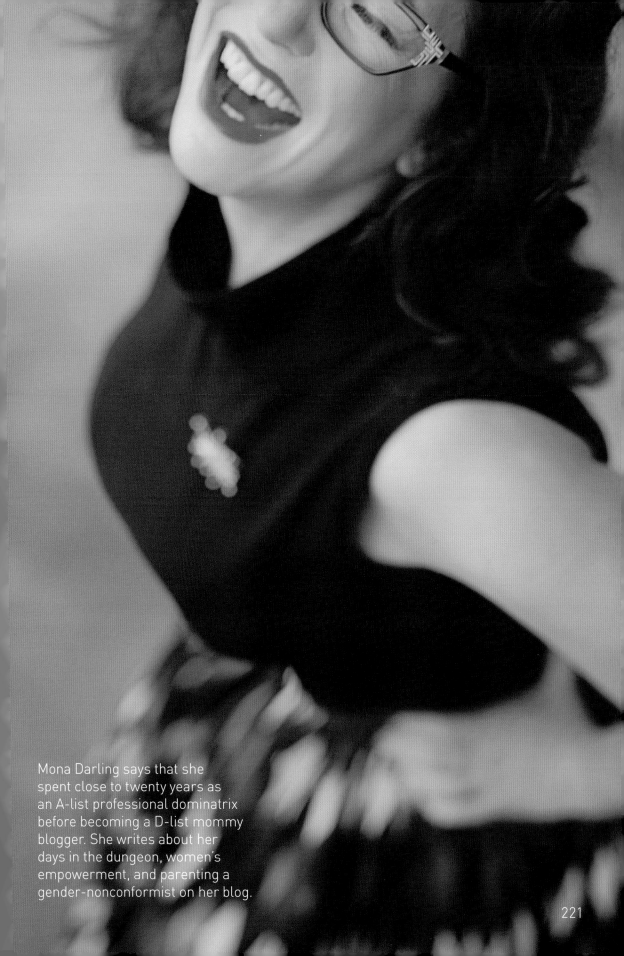

Mona Darling says that she spent close to twenty years as an A-list professional dominatrix before becoming a D-list mommy blogger. She writes about her days in the dungeon, women's empowerment, and parenting a gender-nonconformist on her blog.

NO EVIL COLLECTION BY PICOBONG

2013
Neoprene, Velcro, feathers
picobong.com

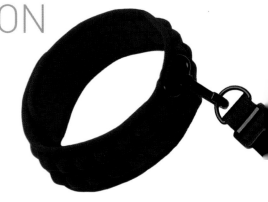

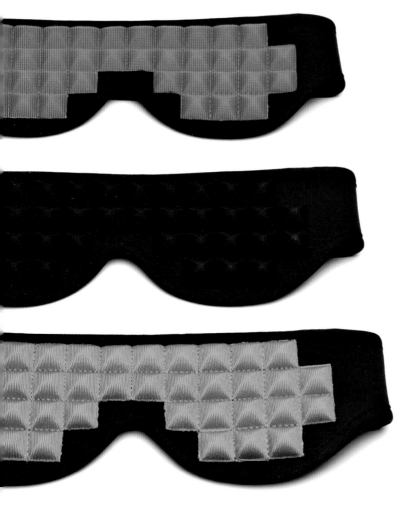

There is something about the act of putting on a blindfold that instantly ups the drama of any kind of experience—think of how exciting it was as a kid to play Pin the Tail on the Donkey or to get your turn to take a blind swing at a piñata. Unlike many other things, the fun of blindfolds doesn't have to stop when you grow up. Part of a collection of light bondage play toys from PicoBong, the See No Evil Blindfold has a soft, retro-futuristic pixelated pattern on the front that would not be out of place in the movie *Tron*. Available in blue, black, and cerise, the machine-washable blindfolds are made with ultra-smooth neoprene and are fastened with Velcro to fit all sizes.

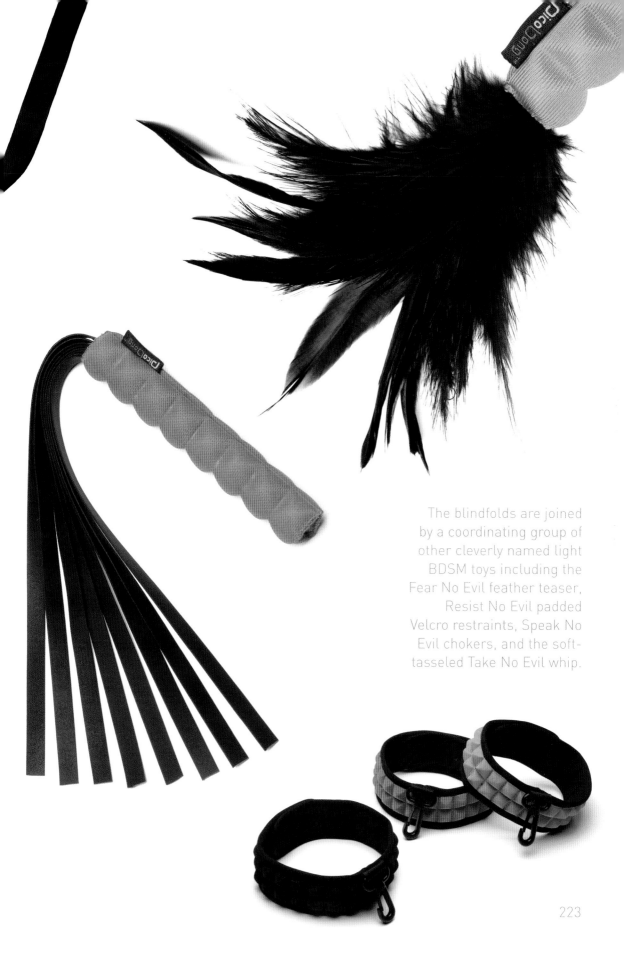

The blindfolds are joined by a coordinating group of other cleverly named light BDSM toys including the Fear No Evil feather teaser, Resist No Evil padded Velcro restraints, Speak No Evil chokers, and the soft-tasseled Take No Evil whip.

LEATHER CUFF BRACELET, LASH BELT, NECKTIE & RAZOR BY INCOQNITO

2009

Stainless steel, base metal, leather, polyester blend, rayon

lovecrave.com

Incoqnito, a line of jewelry and accessories designed by Ii Chang to have a sophisticated, kinky edge, has now become part of Crave. Pieces still in production include the Droplet necklace (page 116), Leather Tassels (page 120), and leather cuffs that can be worn stacked as bracelets or used as handcuffs for light play.

The Lash Belt.

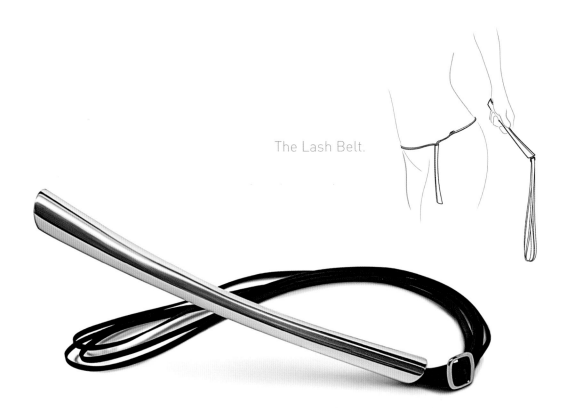

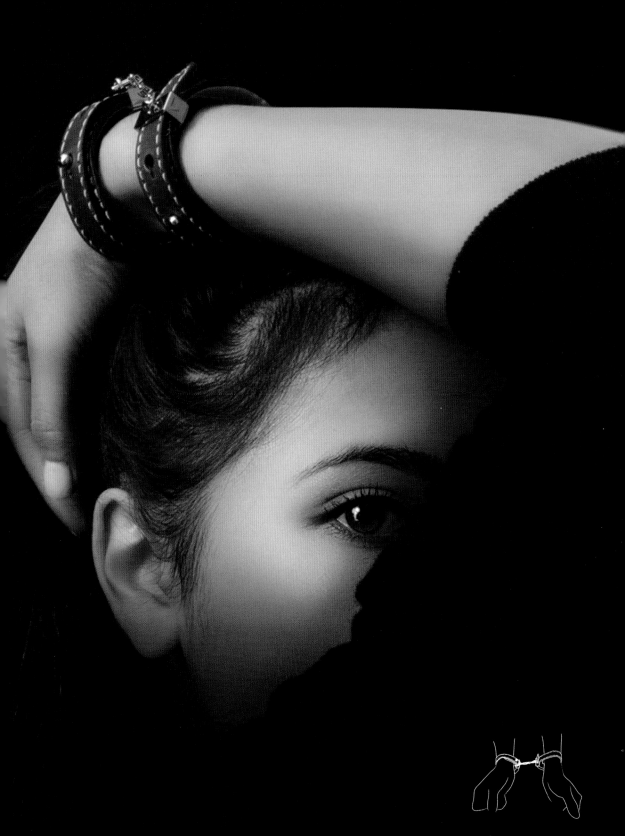

Genuine leather
cuff bracelets.

Discontinued pieces include the adjustable Lash Belt, which transforms into a leather whip, a Necktie accessory that can also be used as an adjustable leash for sensual control of your partner, and the Razor sensation toy that features both a claw and a pinwheel to create a variety of sensations depending on the pressure applied.

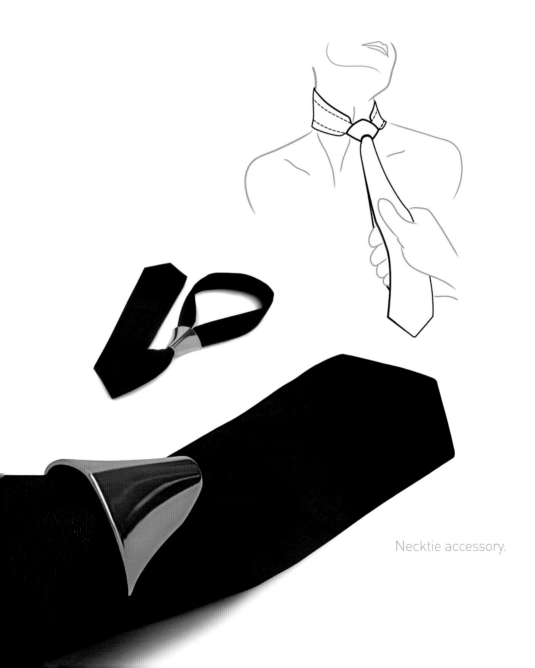

Necktie accessory.

Razor sensation toy.

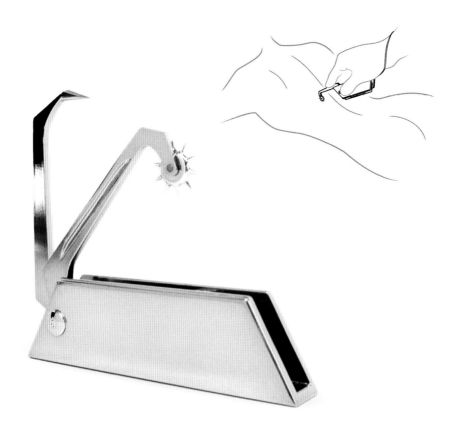

SEDUCE ME COLLECTION
BY JIMMYJANE

2014
Lambskin leather, natural ostrich feathers, glass
jimmyjane.com

Known for its award-winning vibrators,
Jimmyjane has entered the luxury fetish
category with Seduce Me, a collection of
light BDSM toys that includes a riding
crop, blindfold, handcuffs, feather tickler,
and black glass Ben Wa balls. The 15"-
long handmade leather riding crop offers
a wrapped handle made of black lambskin
leather over a fiberglass core, while the
leather blindfold features metal accents
and a gentle elastic band.

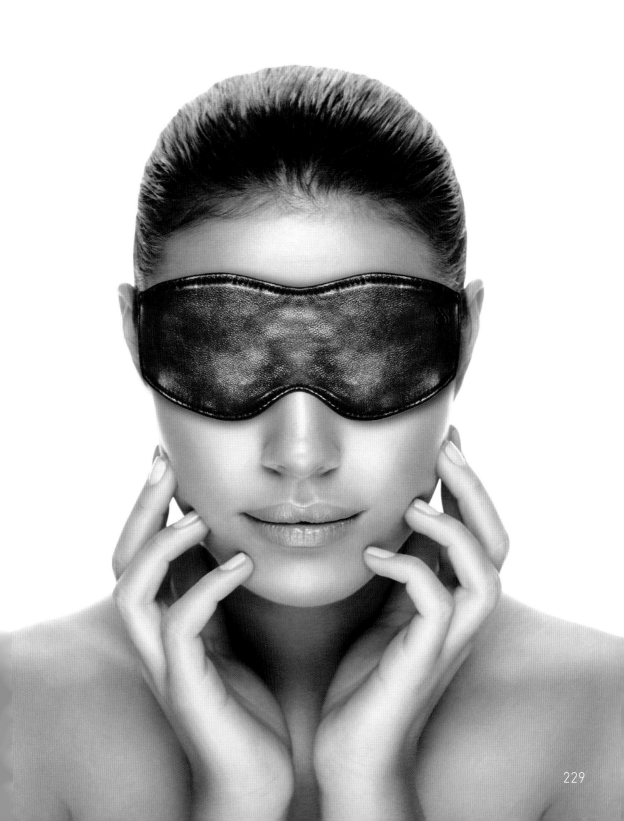

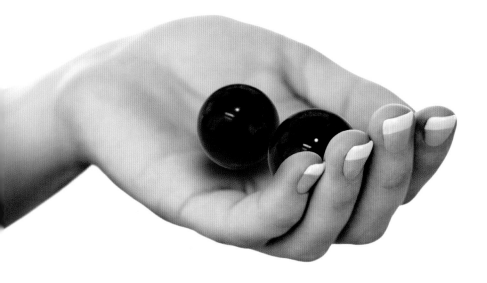

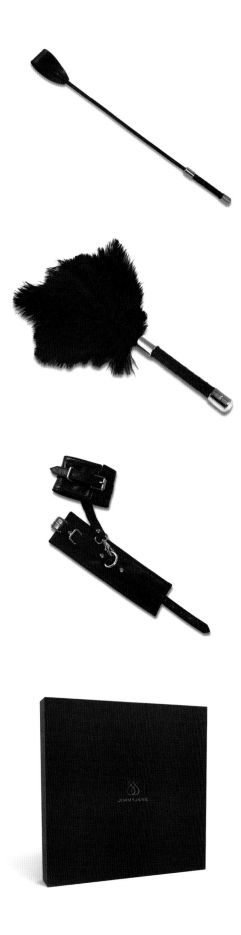

The tickler is made of natural ostrich feathers and a leather-wrapped handle, and leather handcuffs come with a detachable metal connector for light bondage play. Women can insert the black glass balls before sex to feel their weight or leave them in during sex for enhanced sensation.

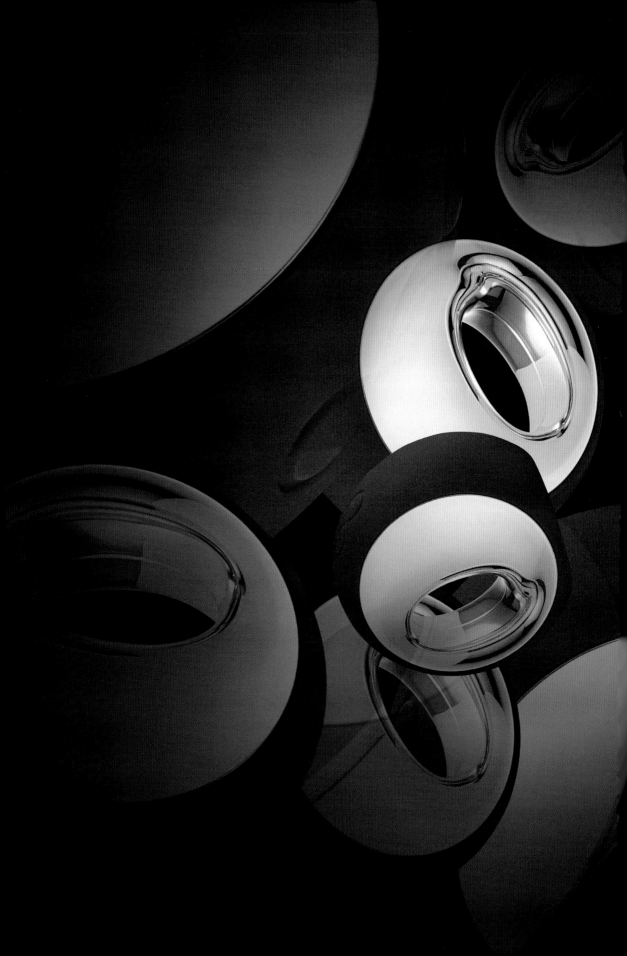

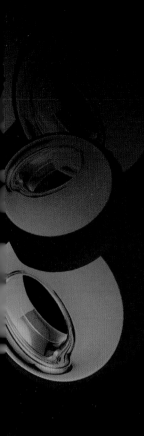

IN A CATEGORY OF THEIR OWN

STRONIC PULSATOR
BY FUN FACTORY

2012 – 2013
Medical-grade silicone
funfactory.com

The Stronic Pulsator is not a dildo or vibrator, but an entirely new type of sex toy. Rather than base all its charm on vibration, this toy uses ten different thrusting rhythms to mimic sexual movements more authentically. It's rather quite startling when you first see it in action, like a disembodied horny member looking for a mate. But this is no novelty toy or gag gift. Stronic is made of medical-grade silicone, is USB-rechargeable and fully submersible, and comes with a two-year full warranty. The 9"-long toy is available in three models: Eins, Zwei, and Drei, all of which can be inserted up to 7 inches. While all can be used vaginally, only Zwei and Drei are recommended for anal use.

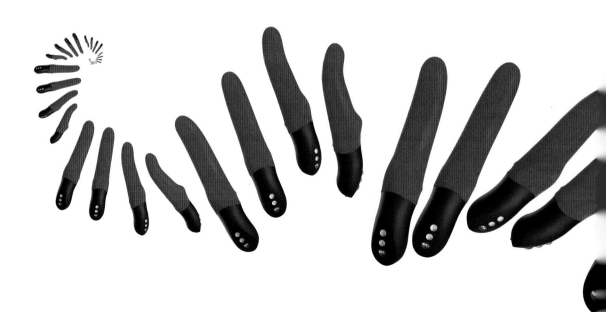

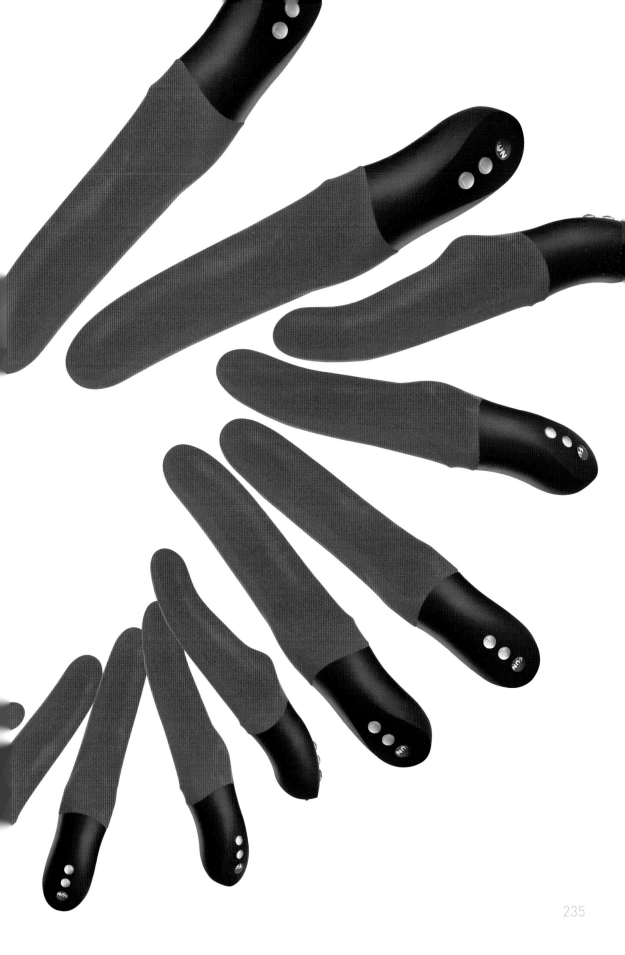

235

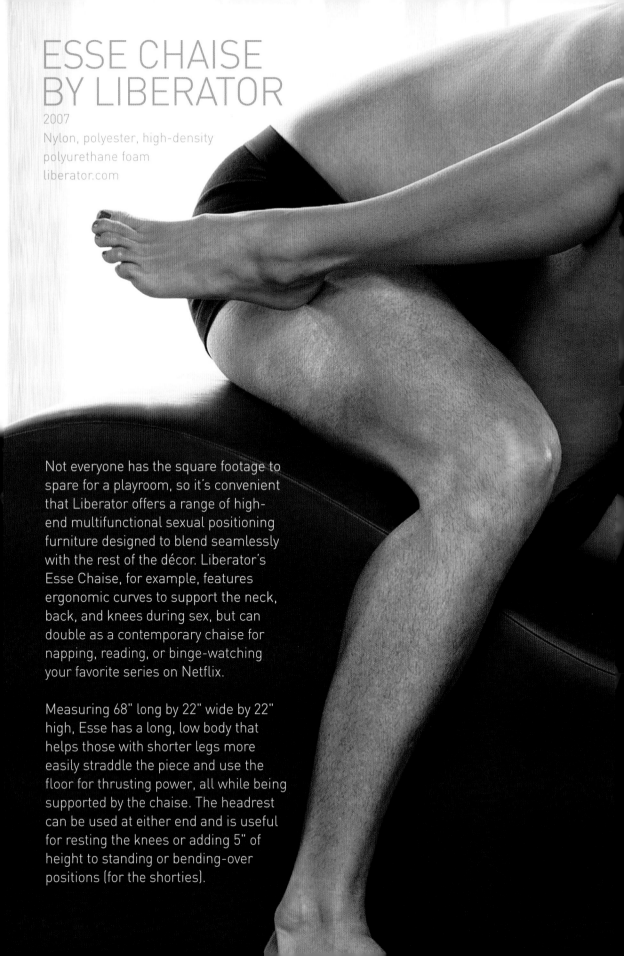

ESSE CHAISE
BY LIBERATOR

2007
Nylon, polyester, high-density
polyurethane foam
liberator.com

Not everyone has the square footage to
spare for a playroom, so it's convenient
that Liberator offers a range of high-
end multifunctional sexual positioning
furniture designed to blend seamlessly
with the rest of the décor. Liberator's
Esse Chaise, for example, features
ergonomic curves to support the neck,
back, and knees during sex, but can
double as a contemporary chaise for
napping, reading, or binge-watching
your favorite series on Netflix.

Measuring 68" long by 22" wide by 22"
high, Esse has a long, low body that
helps those with shorter legs more
easily straddle the piece and use the
floor for thrusting power, all while being
supported by the chaise. The headrest
can be used at either end and is useful
for resting the knees or adding 5" of
height to standing or bending-over
positions (for the shorties).

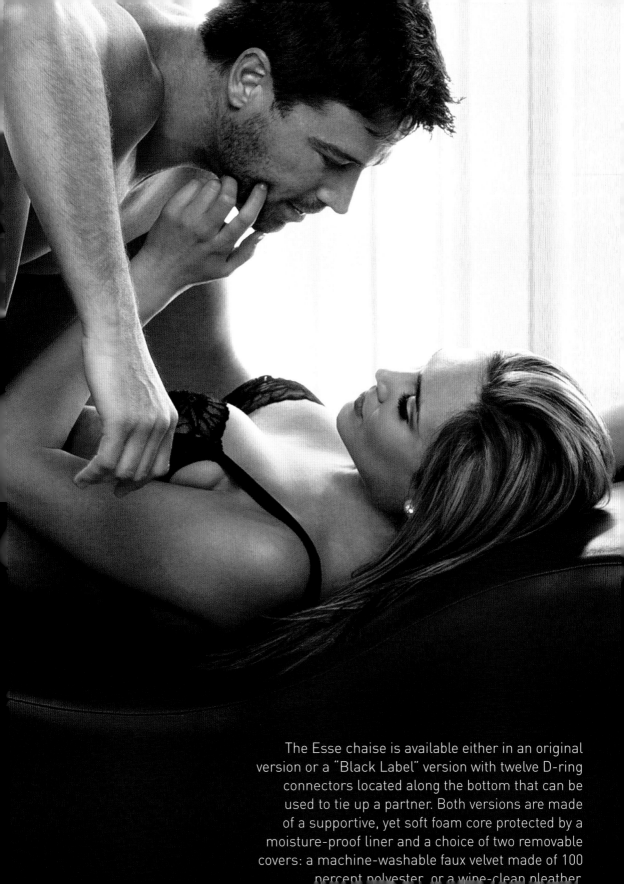

The Esse chaise is available either in an original version or a "Black Label" version with twelve D-ring connectors located along the bottom that can be used to tie up a partner. Both versions are made of a supportive, yet soft foam core protected by a moisture-proof liner and a choice of two removable covers: a machine-washable faux velvet made of 100 percent polyester, or a wipe-clean pleather

ORA 2 ORAL SEX SIMULATOR BY LELO

2014
Body-safe silicone, ABS plastic
lelo.com

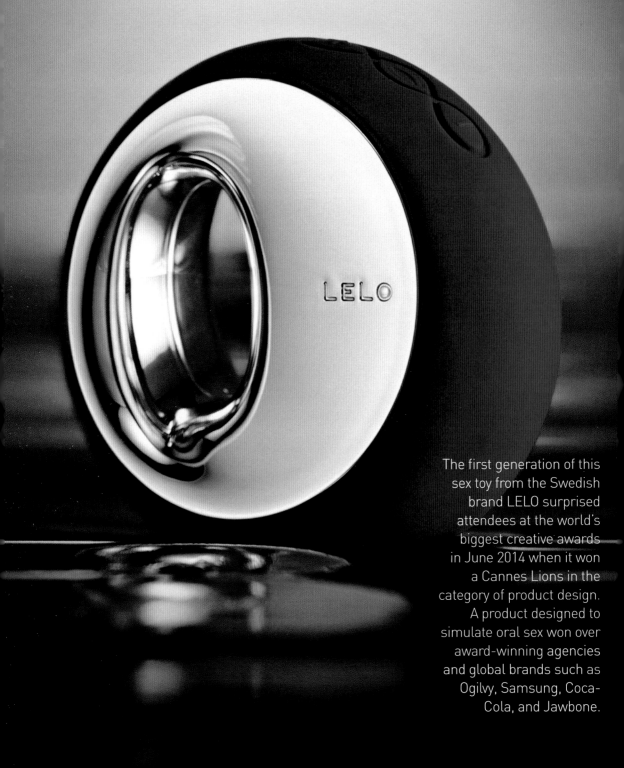

The first generation of this sex toy from the Swedish brand LELO surprised attendees at the world's biggest creative awards in June 2014 when it won a Cannes Lions in the category of product design. A product designed to simulate oral sex won over award-winning agencies and global brands such as Ogilvy, Samsung, Coca-Cola, and Jawbone.

The upgraded ORA 2 combines vibrations with swirling and flicking movements from an enlarged rotating "nub" (which doubles as a tongue) that is concealed underneath a layer of smooth silicone skin. Watching the massaging movement is mesmerizing, like a hypnotist swaying a gold watch before your eyes. For use on and around the clitoris, ORA 2 is waterproof, USB-rechargeable, and offers ten different stimulation patterns that increase in intensity as pressure is applied to the body.

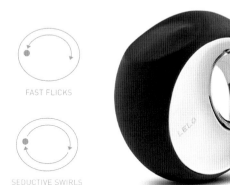

FAST FLICKS

SEDUCTIVE SWIRLS

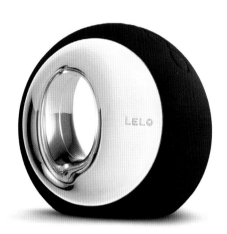

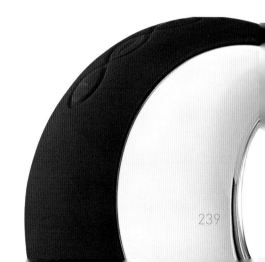

CONDOMS
BY SIR RICHARD'S
CONDOM COMPANY

2011
100% natural filler-free latex, silicone lubricant, foil wrapper
sirrichards.com

Founded in Boulder, Colorado,
by a team of socially conscious
entrepreneurs and designers, Sir
Richard's Condom Company has
donated millions of condoms as
part of their Buy One, Give One
program. Sir Richard's is also
the exclusive condom partner
of (RED), with 5 percent of the
proceeds from every Sir Richard's
(PRODUCT) RED Special Edition
box going to the fight against AIDS.

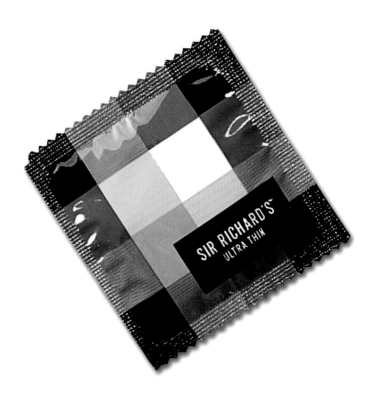

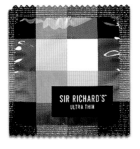
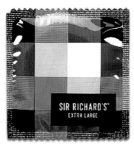
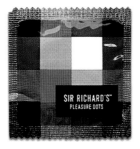
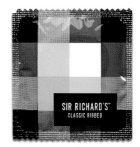
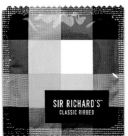
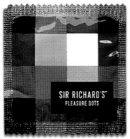
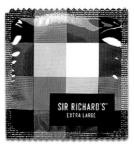
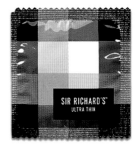
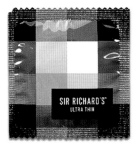
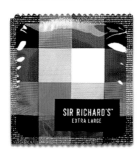
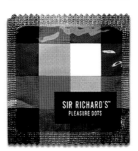
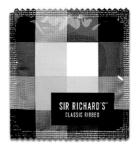
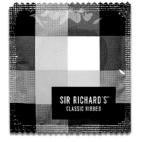
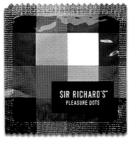

Beyond their charitable endeavors,
Sir Richard's manufactures premium
condoms that are PETA-approved,
vegan-certified, and free of chemicals
like glycerin, parabens, and spermicides.
The packaging colors represent the
various condom types, including Ultra
Thin, Pleasure Dots, Classic Ribbed,
and others. Sir Richard's packaging,
designed by the fully integrated creative
agency TDA_Boulder, uses a simple but
elegant plaid pattern with grayscale
accents for the condom wrapper, box,
and all other brand identity.

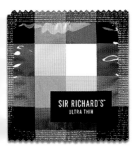
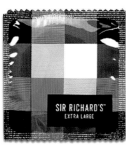

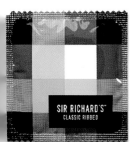
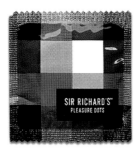
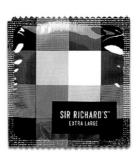
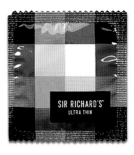

SEMENETTE
BY BERMAN INNOVATIONS LLC

2013
Medical-grade silicone
thesemenette.com

When Stephanie Berman and her wife decided
to conceive a child, they wanted to do it in the
privacy of their own home with the same intimacy
experienced by heterosexual couples. The
only problem was finding a product that could
seamlessly be a part of their lovemaking and also
be used for insemination. Sensing a need in the
market, Berman decided to create something
herself, and the Semenette was born.

The award-winning novelty product is an
anatomically correct dildo with a specially designed
inner tubing and attached pump intended to
mimic ejaculation. Unlike other semen-delivering
methods (turkey basters being the most famous
example), Semenette offers the ability to replace
the embedded plastic tubing with each use,
eliminating sanitary concerns. It also offers the
added benefit of helping to bring the woman to
orgasm, which studies have shown can assist in
successful pregnancies.

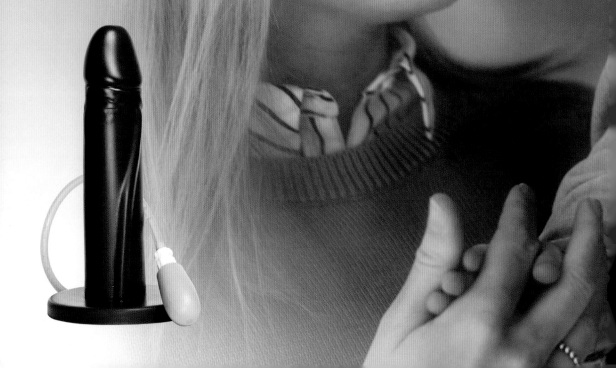

Since it fits into most harnesses, Semenette is also an option for the transgender community, specifically FTM (female-to-male) individuals. Whether used for insemination or just to mimic traditional ejaculation, it allows both partners to enjoy an authentic experience. It can also be helpful for heterosexual couples where the male partner is experiencing erectile issues, serodiscordant couples (where one or both partners are HIV+), fetish or kink groups during adult play, or even adult performers looking for an ejaculating toy for a show.

Made in the US, Semenette comes in one standard 6.25"-long size in vanilla, caramel, and chocolate hues. Berman herself is proof it works—she and her wife successfully used the product to conceive a daughter.

Q&A
THOMAS SANCELOT
FOUNDER
SEXSHOP3D

What inspired you to create SexShop3D? Is your background in sex toy design or 3D printing?
I have never worked for the sex toy or 3D printing industry but I have a passion for new technologies. I work in web design and I saw a 3D printer at a client's house one day. He showed me what he could do with it, and I was hooked instantly. I wondered how I could be a part of the revolution and I realized pretty quickly the sex toy industry was bound to change. Privacy, convenience, customization, and cost are key factors when getting a sex toy. That's what 3D printing offers.

How many players are in the 3D sex toy market at the moment?
SexShop3D is the only company selling 3D sex toy designs. You must realize that even though 3D printing is a thirty-year-old technology, it really took off in the last few years with the maker movement driven by hobbyists and the open source philosophy. We are the first attempt to monetize the concept of 3D printing sex toys at home. A company is selling 3D-printed sex toys as finished products but we believe the revolution in the sex toy industry will come from the fact that home 3D printing eliminates the manufacturing step between sellers and consumers.

What is the main reason you think people are interested in this technology?
When you own a 3D printer, you want the ability to print as many things as possible. Why not sex toys? It can be done instantly from home. Nobody knows what you are using your 3D printer for. You simply get a 3D model from our website and you can print a sex toy in the size and material you want. It can be hard or flexible plastic, for example, and in the color of your choice. A 3D printer comes at a cost of course, but printing a sex toy will cost you around $10 including the price to get the design from us.

What type of material do you recommend for the printing?
In home 3D printing, you mainly print in plastic. You have a choice between PLA and ABS plastic. We recommend printing your sex toys with ABS. The part can be easily smoothed, and it is totally body safe. We also recommend spraying your sex toy with thin coats of silicone. ABS plastic and silicone are common materials in traditional sex toys, and they are the preferred materials for 3D printed sex toys, too.

Do you know anything about your typical customer?
Eighty percent of our customers are men but this technology is so new that I am sure it will even up when home 3D printers become more common. Recently on my blog, a couple that had just bought a 3D printer on Cyber Monday asked me about 3D printed sex toys admitting being "new to the 3D printing world." Our typical customer is not different from those of traditional sex shops; he just owns a 3D printer.

What has been the biggest challenge for printing 3D sex toys at home?
We were able to introduce methods to print sex toys in silicone and that was our biggest achievement in the safety department. Now we could actually say that 3D printing our own sex toys is also safer. Did you know the sex toy industry is not regulated? Sex toys are "novelty items" for a "novelty use" so there aren't any hygiene or safety standards. By making them yourself on a 3D printer you can choose to use proper body-safe materials.

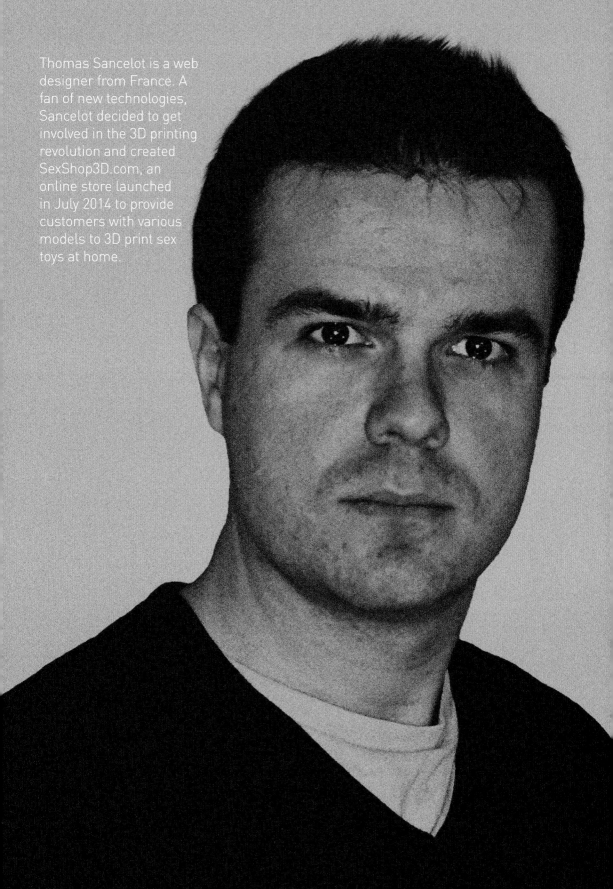

Thomas Sancelot is a web designer from France. A fan of new technologies, Sancelot decided to get involved in the 3D printing revolution and created SexShop3D.com, an online store launched in July 2014 to provide customers with various models to 3D print sex toys at home.

The most popular SexShop3D model is shown here on an Ultimaker 2 digital printer. The realistic dildo takes about eight hours to print and represents a third of all sales for the company.

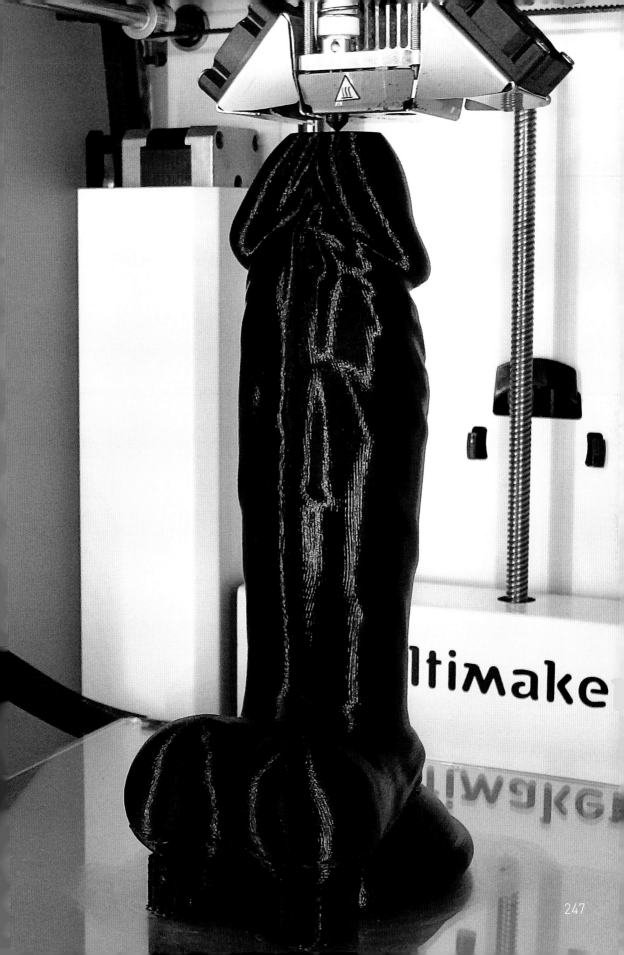

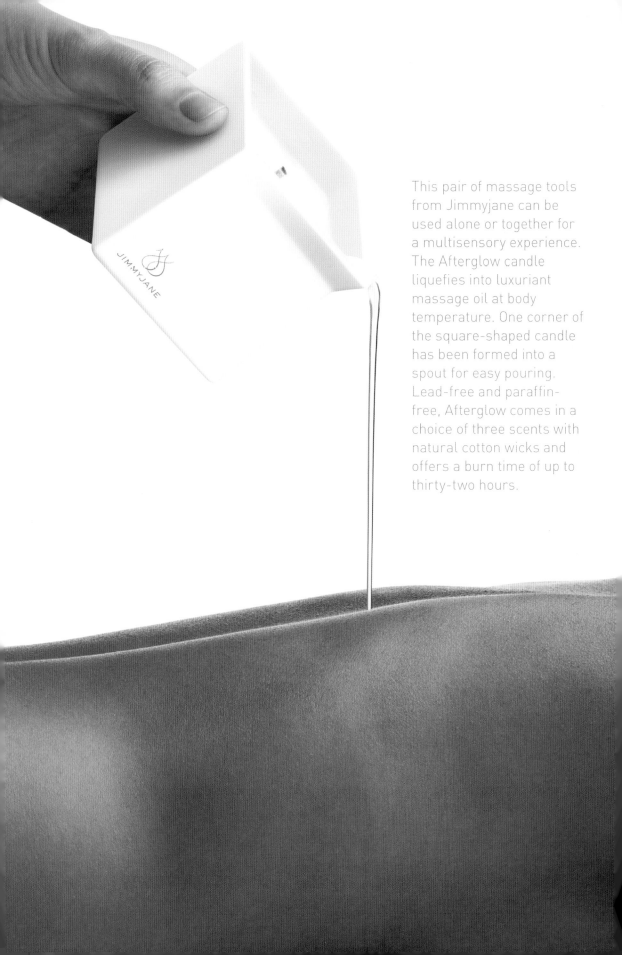

This pair of massage tools from Jimmyjane can be used alone or together for a multisensory experience. The Afterglow candle liquefies into luxuriant massage oil at body temperature. One corner of the square-shaped candle has been formed into a spout for easy pouring. Lead-free and paraffin-free, Afterglow comes in a choice of three scents with natural cotton wicks and offers a burn time of up to thirty-two hours.

CONTOUR M MASSAGE STONE & AFTERGLOW MASSAGE OIL CANDLE BY JIMMYJANE

2008

Porcelain (Contour M), jojoba, shea butter, Vitamin E, soy, aloe (candle), ceramic (candle holder)

jimmyjane.com

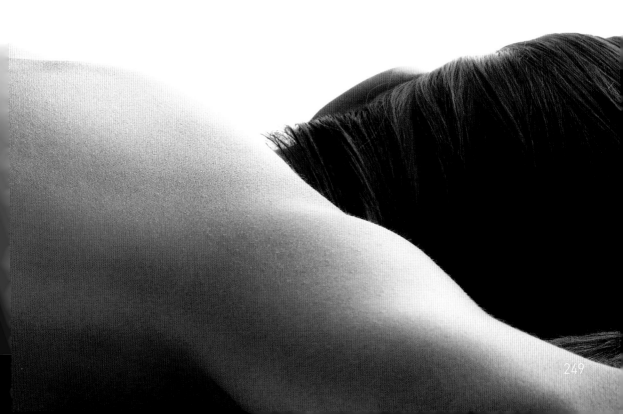

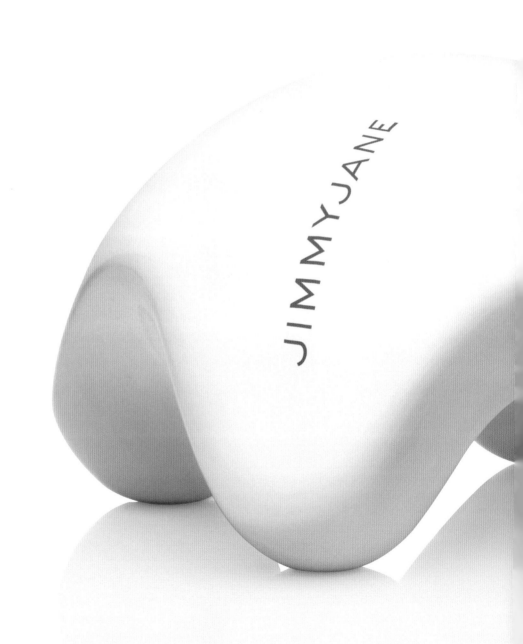

The IDEA Award-winning Contour massage stone can be warmed up for a soothing experience or cooled down for a refreshing one. Its smooth, polished surface of double-fired porcelain easily glides over the skin; the large dome can be used for large strokes while the four small nodes offer multipoint stimulation.

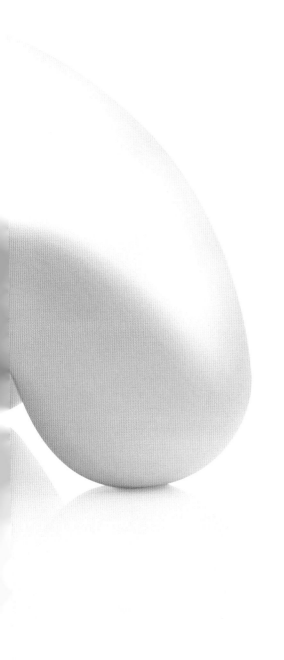

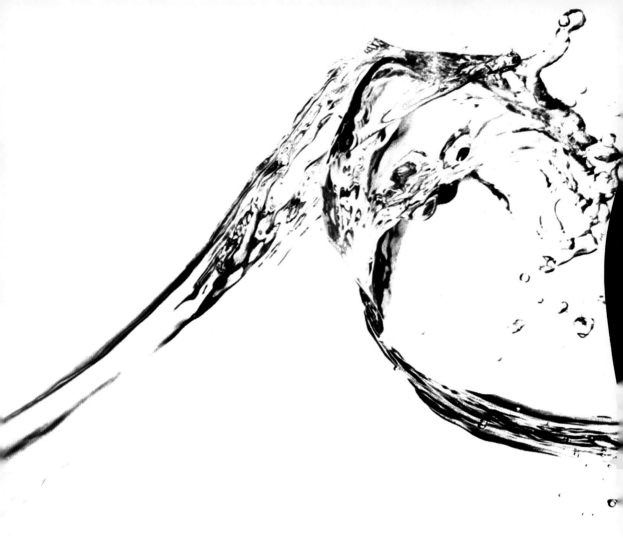

H20 VIBE
BY DROP OF SWEDEN
2014
Medical-grade silicone, ABS plastic
dropofsweden.se

Although women have been using water pressure to get off
in the bathroom since hand showers were first invented,
the Scandinavian designers behind Drop of Sweden have
taken things a step further with the H20 Vibe. This 100
percent waterproof hybrid toy combines an insertable
vibrator with an adjustable silicone nozzle that directs a
stream of water towards the clitoris. Designed to attach to
99 percent of standard shower hose connectors, the toy's
water jet intensity and temperature are adjusted by the
main shower controls.

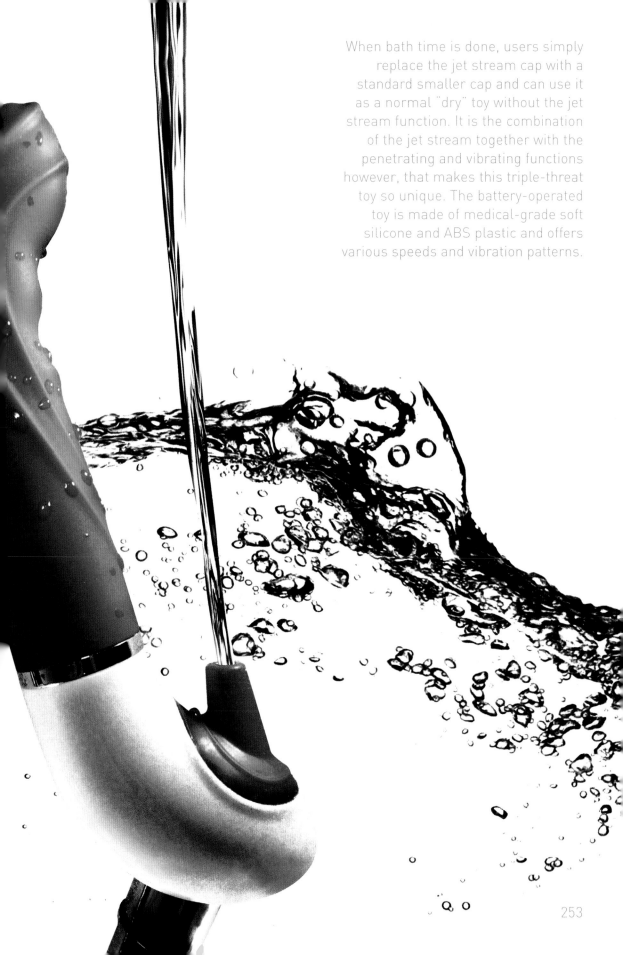

When bath time is done, users simply replace the jet stream cap with a standard smaller cap and can use it as a normal "dry" toy without the jet stream function. It is the combination of the jet stream together with the penetrating and vibrating functions however, that makes this triple-threat toy so unique. The battery-operated toy is made of medical-grade soft silicone and ABS plastic and offers various speeds and vibration patterns.

253

TRANSFORMER
BY PICOBONG

2014
Body-safe, FDA-approved silicone
picobong.com

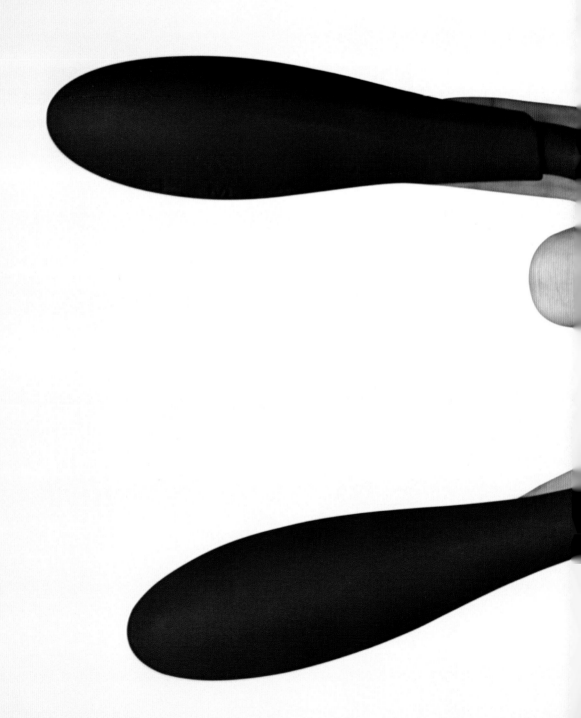

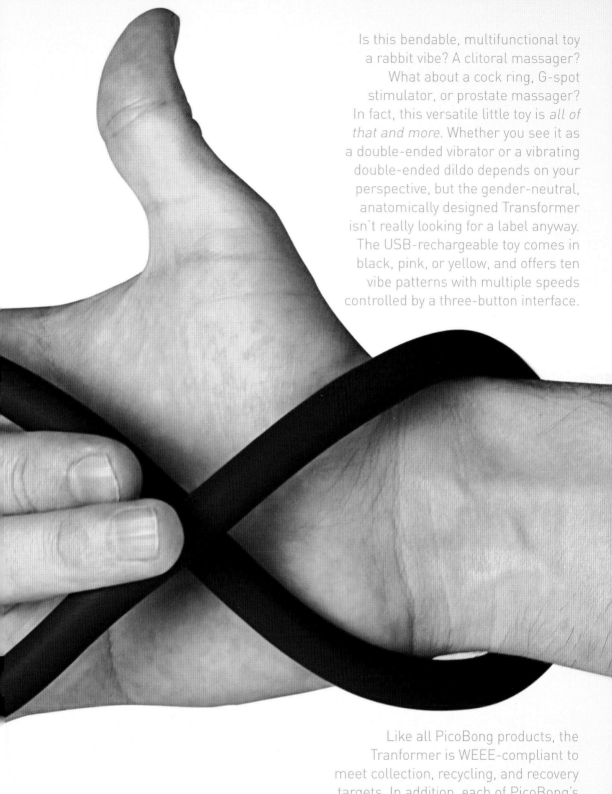

Is this bendable, multifunctional toy a rabbit vibe? A clitoral massager? What about a cock ring, G-spot stimulator, or prostate massager? In fact, this versatile little toy is *all of that and more*. Whether you see it as a double-ended vibrator or a vibrating double-ended dildo depends on your perspective, but the gender-neutral, anatomically designed Transformer isn't really looking for a label anyway. The USB-rechargeable toy comes in black, pink, or yellow, and offers ten vibe patterns with multiple speeds controlled by a three-button interface.

Like all PicoBong products, the Tranformer is WEEE-compliant to meet collection, recycling, and recovery targets. In addition, each of PicoBong's manufacturing facilities follows ISO standards of quality management to ensure quality output and increased efficiency.

CONDOMS
BY NAKED CONDOMS

2010
Latex, silicone lubricant, foil wrapper
nakedcondoms.com

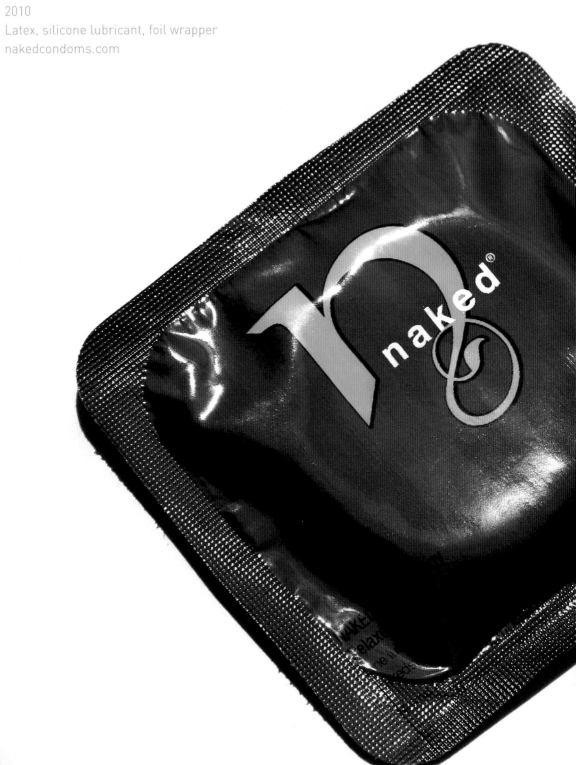

These luxury condoms made the news for earning a coveted spot in the 2015 Oscar swag bag. Each sleek rectangular box slides open to showcase six condoms in bright wrappers that indicate size by color. These condoms are more than just a pretty package however. Available in four sizes (from Tight to X Large), Naked's condoms are designed with a patented Pleasure Fit shape that enhances sensitivity. Dipped from soft, thin latex, the condoms are covered with a thin layer of high-quality silicone lubricant specially formulated for use with the product.

According to Jacob Tempchin, Operations & Sales for Naked Condoms, the company has a mission to make condoms sexier as well as a strong commitment to family planning. "Our mission is to give women a product to empower themselves sexually," says Tempchin. With the help of the Global Poverty Project, Naked Condoms has committed to provide two million condoms to the country of Uganda, and 20 percent of all future company profits will be donated to organizations furthering access to international family planning and global health initiatives.

COMING CANDLE BY HEFF

2015
Pigmented concrete
heff.nyc

HEFF is a contemporary art practice in Brooklyn, New York, that explores the territories between art and design, from small objects to large public works. The studio sells sculptural designs in limited product runs, with two new objects released each month. Made of pigmented concrete, the Coming Candle features a pair of spheres that support a 6 ½" candle within a friction-fit tapered shaft—when the candle is lit, the melting wax creates a symbolic "release." The 1.5" x 2.5" x 1.75" candle holder is designed for use with any tapered candle with a diameter from ½"' to ¾". While intended as a table decoration, if dinner goes well, the candle could also find a place in the bedroom. It is generally recommended to use plain, 100 percent paraffin candles with any wax play as they burn at a safer temperature.

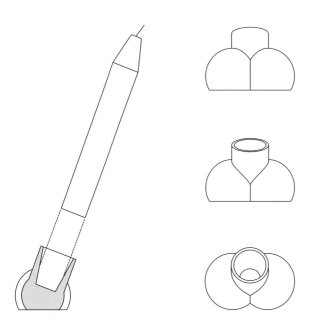

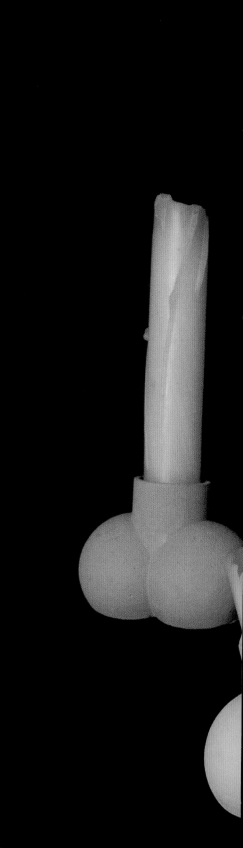

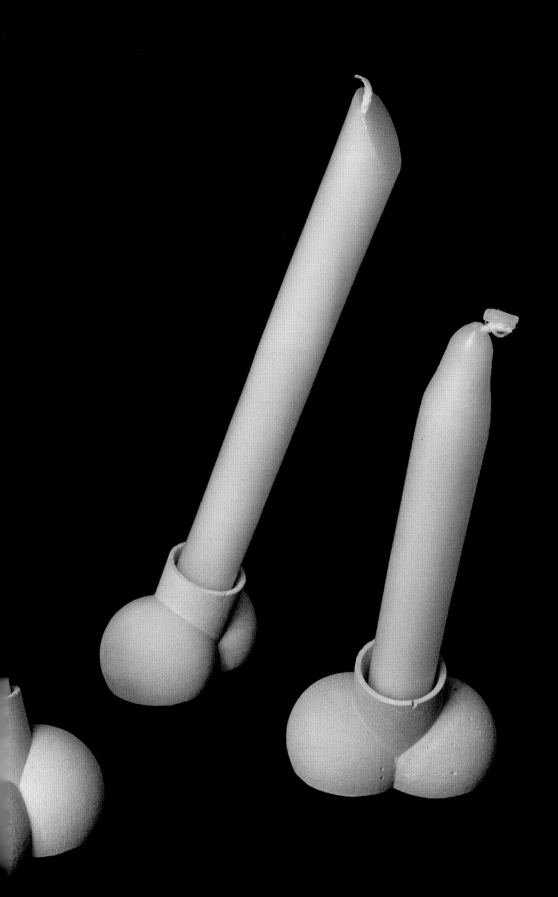

SALì CHAISE & SECRET CUSHION BY MÉNAGE À QUATRE

2014, 2013
Hard maple, foam, upholstery (Salì);
fabric, down, foam (Secret Cushion)
menageaquatre.net

Created for an off-site event held during Milan Design Week 2014, these prototypes are intended to help make the process of experimenting with different sexual positions more comfortable. Created in collaboration with Vincent Joseph Monastero, Matthew Alexander Cherkas, and Viviane Yazdani, Salì is a four-legged seat with a cushion "saddle" that encourages partners to explore new sexual positions, particularly those standing up. Measuring 22" wide, 22" long, and 34" high, Salì has a discreet design that belies its real purpose.

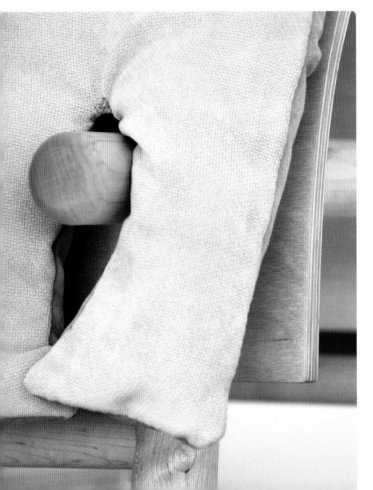

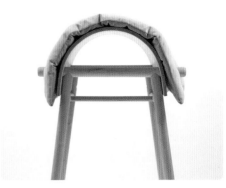

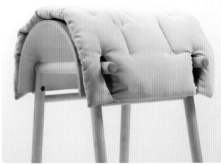

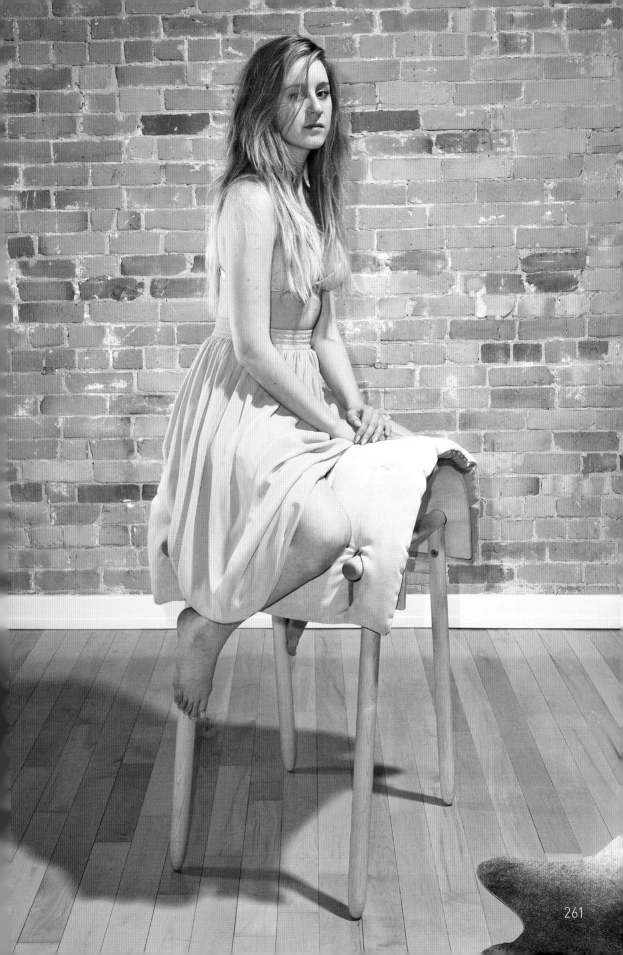

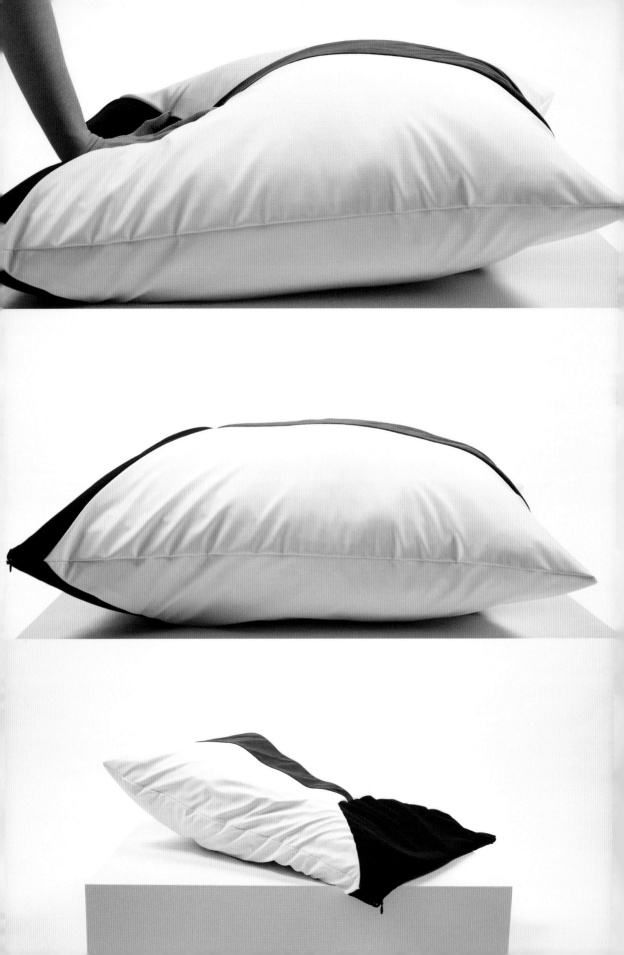

Secret Cushion, a collaboration between Yazdani and Alisa Maria Wronski, is a soft pillow designed to help support the body, enhance angles, and alleviate stress during different positions of sexual intercourse. The supporting wedge-shaped material is disguised in a soft cover so that when pressure is applied it compresses and holds its shape. The cushion regains its shape in a few minutes, helping to keep your secrets intact.

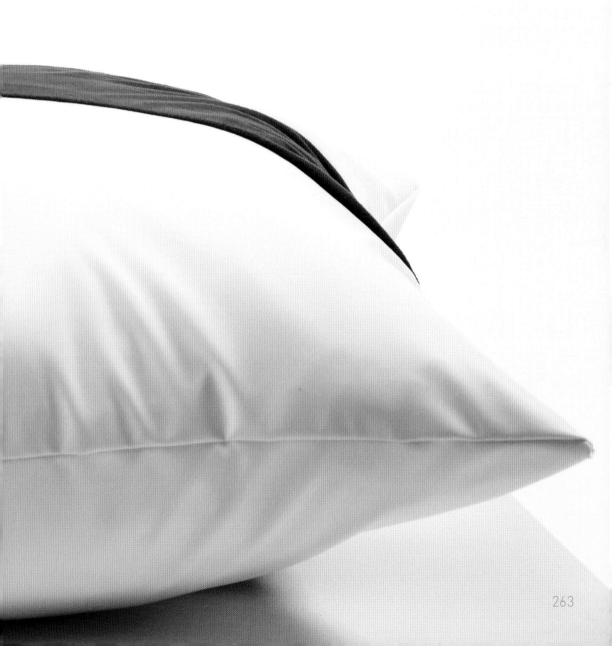

WHERE TO GET IT

There are plenty of virtual and physical shops to purchase these products safely and discreetly. Many manufacturers and designers also sell directly from their own sites. Shop around a bit online to try to get the best price, but make sure the sites are reputable and have secure payment systems. If you need advice, don't be afraid to ask—customer service lines and shops are staffed with highly informed salespeople who are there to help.

Adam & Eve
Adameve.com
Around for forty years, Adam & Eve is a leading adult toys company in the US. This online superstore sells erotic toys and movies for gays, straights, and everyone in between.

AHAnoir
Ahanoir.com
The sister site to AHAlife, AHAnoir is an upscale site for higher-end erotic toys, apparel, and accessories.

Babeland
babeland.com
Founded in 1993 by Claire Cavanah and Rachel Venning, Babeland has shops in New York City and Seattle and an online shop with incredibly helpful user reviews.

Come As You Are Co-Operative
comeasyouare.com
This Toronto-based retailer claims to be the world's only worker-owned co-operative sex shop; they don't make commission or profit from customer purchases.

Early To Bed
Early2bed.com
Early to Bed opened in September 2001 on Chicago's north side when owner Searah Deysach felt the city needed a place where women (and people of all genders) could shop for quality sex toys in a safe, welcoming space.

Eve's Garden
evesgarden.com
Founded in 1974 by the late women's rights activist Dell Williams, Eve's Garden is the world's first mail-order catalog and sexuality boutique designed for the unique needs of women. Visitors can shop online or at the New York City store.

Good Vibrations
goodvibes.com
With shops in San Francisco and Berkeley, Good Vibrations has been promoting sexual health and pleasure since 1977. Shoppers can buy sex toys, books, and movies, and attend workshops.

LeLuv
leluv.com
This online retailer offers free shipping in the United States.

Lovehoney
lovehoney.co.uk
The UK's biggest online adult retailer claims that one in three sex toys sold in the UK comes from their warehouse in Bath, England.

Peekay
peekay.com
Peekay, Inc. is an award-winning specialty retailer with an emphasis on lingerie and sexual health and wellness products. The company operates forty-five stores in six states, under the Lovers, A Touch of Romance, ConRev, and Christal's brands.

She Bop
sheboptheshop.com
Evy Cowan and Jeneen Doumitt opened She Bop in November of 2009 with the objective of creating an adult boutique specializing in non-toxic, body-safe toys, exceptional books, female- and queer-friendly DVDs, and quality sensuality products. There are now two shops in Portland and an online store.

SheVibe
shevibe.com
This comprehensive shopping site includes original artwork, weekly discounts, flash sales, and one of the best customer review programs in the industry.

The Pleasure Chest
thepleasurechest.com
The Pleasure Chest started in 1971 in the West Village in New York City at the height of the sexual revolution and currently has shops in Chicago, Los Angeles, and New York City.

RESOURCES

Some helpful sources for more information on erotic objects and sexuality in general.

CENTERS & MUSEUMS

Center for Sex & Culture
San Francisco
sexandculture.org
The mission of the Center for Sex & Culture is to provide judgment-free education, cultural events, a library/media archive, and other resources to audiences across the sexual and gender spectrum. The center also researches and disseminates factual information, framing and informing issues of public policy and public health.

Museum of Sex
New York City
museumofsex.com
The goal of the Museum of Sex is to preserve and present the history, evolution, and cultural significance of human sexuality. The museum produces exhibitions, publications, and programs that bring the best of current scholarship on sex and sexuality to the widest possible audience and is committed to encouraging public enlightenment, discourse, and engagement.

Good Vibrations' Antique Vibrator Museum
San Francisco
antiquevibratormuseum.com
Good Vibrations's founder Joani Blank collected antique vibrators for more than twenty years, and this collection includes her finds as well as those donated by customers who find them at flea markets and through their relatives' estates. The vibes in the collection date from the late 1800s up through the 1970s, and include dozens of styles of electric vibrators that were available to medical professionals and then home consumers. Lead by staff sexologist Dr. Carol Queen, Antique Vibrator History Tours cover the invention and functions of early vibrators.

The Erotic Heritage Museum
Las Vegas
eroticheritagemuseumlasvegas.com
The Harry Mohney Erotic Museum, also known as the Erotic Heritage Museum, was originally created as a partnership between a preacher and a pornographer. Rev. Ted McIlvenna and Harry Mohney agreed to work together to create the Las Vegas Erotic Heritage Museum and maintain a mission of preservation of erotic artifacts, fine art, and film.

The Center for Sexual Pleasure & Health
Pawtucket, Rhode Island
thecsph.org
The Center for Sexual Pleasure & Health is a sexuality education and training organization that works to reduce sexual shame, challenge misinformation, and advance the field of sexuality. It provides professional training, educational initiatives, and community events to help create a more sexually literate society and promote sexual health and wellness.

CONFERENCES + EXPOS

Adult Novelty Manufacturers Expo (ANME)
anmefounders.com
A trade show event for US- and Canadian-based manufacturers to showcase and sell their products to distributor and retailer buyers.

AVN Adult Novelty Expo
noveltyexpo.com
The world's largest adult entertainment expo, held annually.

CatalystCon
catalystcon.com
CatalystCon is a conference created to inspire conversations about sexuality and change how society talks about and treats sexuality.

Sexual Health Expo (SHE)
sexualhealthexpo.com
SHE is intended to connect the general public with professionals to openly explore sexual wellness. Past events have been held in Los Angeles and New York City.

BLOGGERS

Cara Sutra
carasutra.co.uk/blog
Cara Sutra is a British-based sex writer who shares sex toy reviews, erotica, and industry news on her award-winning sex blog.

Dangerous Lilly
dangerouslilly.com/sex-toy-reviews
On her blog, Lilly writes honest reviews on sex toys, offers an informative sex toy care and cleaning guide, and promotes body-safe toys.

Ducky Doolittle
blog.duckydoolittle.com
Writer, speaker, and educator Ducky Doolittle writes about sex toys, safe sex, and sex education at this bright and welcoming site.

Gritty Woman
thegrittywoman.com
Gritty Woman shares her erotic photography and stories, in-depth sex toy reviews, educational guides, and her personal experiences on sex, body positivity, BDSM, and kink on this sex blog.

Hey Epiphora!
heyepiphora.com
For her popular blog, Epiphora tests sex toys and writes up honest sex toy reviews, matter-of-fact masturbation journals, industry critiques, and sex blogging tips.

Kink and Code
kinkandcode.com
This sex-positive hub for technology, dating, sex, and relationships, includes reviews of apps, sites, and toys by freelance writer Emma McGowan.

Lauren Marie Fleming
laurenmariefleming.com
On her site Fleming, a.k.a. Queerie Bradshaw, writes about self-image, relationships, and sex.

Lorax of Sex
loraxofsex.com
This Seattle-based blogger reviews toys and educates readers on sexual health, kink, and other subjects.

Minxy Milly
minxymilly.com
Milly reviews sex toys and writes about dating and relationships on her smart and helpful site.

Naughty Reenie
naughtyreenie.com
Reenie might be naughty, but she is quite good at thoroughly testing and reviewing sex toys on her new site.

Property of Potter
propertyofpotter.com
"Potter" is a twenty-something New England-based mom who launched this blog in 2013 to review sex toys and share other personal thoughts, including poetry.

Searah's Museum of Screwy Sex Toys
screwysextoys.com
This fun site by the owner of the Chicago-based sex toy shop Early to Bed takes a irreverent look at funny, unusual, and "scary" sex toys.

The Adventures of Mona Darling
darlingpropaganda.com
Mona Darling says that she spent close to twenty years as an A-list professional dominatrix before becoming a D-list mommy blogger. She writes about her days in the dungeon, women's empowerment, and parenting a gender-nonconformist.

The Redhead Bedhead
redheadbedhead.com
A writer, educator, and adult retail consultant, JoEllen Notte reviews sex toys and writes about sexual health, relationships, and trends on this blog where her goal is "saving the world from mediocre sex."

Continued on next page

RESOURCES

OTHER ONLINE SOURCES

Dildo Generator
dildo-generator.com
This online DIY tool lets you easily design your own dildo, then save and export the file to be used with a 3D printer.

Dildology.org
dildology.org
This much-needed site, which has the motto *In Dildo Veritas*, intends to provide material verification services and maintain a public database of the results, adding transparency and oversight to the industry while educating the public about the science behind pleasure products.

Frisky Feminist Press
friskyfeminist.com
Run by Lauren Marie Fleming, this site is dedicated to providing accessible, judgment-free, comprehensive sex education.

Future of Sex
futureofsex.net
Future of Sex provides insights into the future of human sex and sexuality by looking at how communication, interface, biological, and other technologies are enabling new expressions of human sexuality. Sections include Virtual Sex, Remote Sex, Immersive Entertainment, Robots, Sex Tech, Augmentation, and Bizarre Bazaar, an eighteen-plus showcase of products and services.

Kinkly
kinkly.com
This site includes a sex toy directory, a list of top sex bloggers, a "sex position playlist," and articles on sexual health and news.

Makerlove
makerlove.com
This site provides free sex toy designs for 3D printers. Users can privately download designs that may be used along with vibrating motors purchased elsewhere. Current designs include butt plugs, dildos, anal beads, and vibrators in various (and sometimes humorous) forms.

Oh Joy Sex Toy
ohjoysextoy.com
A weekly, eighteen-and-over web comic by Erika Moen that reviews everything related to sex and the sex industry—from toys to positions to sexual health and the roles of sex industry workers—in a fun, friendly, and informative way.

Slutty Girl Problems
sluttygirlproblems.com
Reclaiming the word *slut* to mean a woman who is empowered by her sexuality, this site is an online community for sex-positive young women. It features humorous columns, sex guides, health and beauty advice, and in-depth sex toy reviews.

Xbiz: The Industry Source
xbiz.com
Adult industry site featuring daily news on web/tech, movie reviews, sex toy reviews, and more.

ACKNOWLEDGMENTS

First of all, thanks to my incredibly talented friend Jason Scuderi for collaborating with me on this project. Without your support, patience, and enthusiasm, this book might still be a pipe dream. Thanks to all of my family and friends for the encouragement to step outside of my comfort zone and never look back. Thanks to Sarah Forbes and Carol Queen for your generous contributions, and to all of the manufacturers, designers, and interview subjects who shared their time and valuable knowledge. I am grateful to Diana Whitney for introducing me to Dede Cummings, our multi-talented literary agent who helped us find a home for the book along with Desmond Peeples. Thanks to Pete Schiffer and everyone at Schiffer Publishing for helping us bring our book to life. Last but not least, a special thanks to my very own object of desire, Stewart, and the two beautiful products of our design.

— Rita Catinella Orrell

A hearty thank-you to the people who made this possible. Rita for bringing me on to this amazing project and allowing me to have a voice. Dede Cummings for her wisdom and help throughout the process, and her assistant, Desmond Peeples, for the hustle behind the scenes. All of the wonderful product designers, manufacturers, and interviewed participants. Schiffer Publishing for believing in this project. And finally, Nami for her patience and understanding for me to see this through.

— Jason Scuderi

PHOTO CREDITS

Cover, front, Michael Topolovac/Crave.
Cover, back, Rosebuds SARL.
We-Vibe 4 Plus, p. 16-17, photo courtesy of We-Vibe.
LYLA 2, p. 18-19, LELO.
Vibease, p. 20-21, Vibease.
Claire Cavanah & Rachel Venning, p. 23, © Sarah Small.
BlueMotion, p. 24-25, OhMiBod.
Lovense Remote Players, p. 26-27, Lovense Product Photos.
Onyx & Pearl, p. 28-29, Kiiroo.com/Amsterdam 2015.
Sarah Forbes, p. 31, Sven Lindahl.
Trainer Toyfriend, p. 34-35, Kjell B. Persson.
Lovelife Kegel Weights, p. 36-37, OhMiBod.
Evi, p. 39, image courtesy of Aneros.
Lauren Marie Fleming, p. 41, Bob Williams.
KGoal, p. 42-43, Minna Life/Makewell.
Jon Millward, p. 45-47, JonMillward.com/blog.
HUM Artificially Intelligent Vibrator, p. 50-51,
J. Dixx Photography (photography),
Dimensional Industries (rendering).
Love the Bird, p. 52-53, photos by Marya Ghazzaoui.
Sono Love, p. 54-55, © Georg Milde.
Mod Open-Source Vibrator, p. 56-57, images courtesy www.comingle.io.
Eric Kalen, p. 59, Andreas Lind.
Pocket & Power Toyfriends, p. 61, Andreas Lind.
Iroha Midori, Sakura & Yuki, p. 63-65, images courtesy of Tenga Co. Ltd.
Smile Makers, p. 66-67, Julian Wolkenstein.
Revel Body SOL, p. 68-69, Revel Body.
Lovelife Collection, p. 70-71, OhMiBod.
Minna Limon, p. 72-73, Brian Krieger/Minna Life.
TARA, p. 74-75, LELO.
SMART WAND, p. 77, LELO.
Molly Murphy, p. 79, Jimmyjane.
FORM Vibrators, p. 80-83, Jimmyjane.
Duet Lux, p. 84-87, Michael Topolovac/Crave.
Vi-Bo Vibrators, p. 88-91, images courtesy Tenga Co. Ltd.
Hello Touch, p. 92-95, Jimmyjane.
INA WAVE, p. 96-97, LELO.
Iroha Mikazuki & Minamo, p. 98-101, images courtesy of Tenga Co. Ltd.
Eva, p. 102-103, David Block (left page), Jeffrey C. Lu (right page),
drawings courtesy Dame Products.
Flex, p. 104-107, Michael Topolovac/Crave.
Whoop.de.doo, p. 108-111, ©annamaresova.com.
Vesper, p. 114-115, Michael Topolovac/Crave.
Droplet, p. 116-117, Michael Topolovac/Crave.
Ti Chang, p. 119, Michael Topolovac/Crave.
Leather Tassels, p. 120-121, Michael Topolovac/Crave.
Ménage à Quatre Rings, p. 122-125,
images courtesy of designer Viviane Yazdani,
© 2013 Ménage à Quatre, all rights reserved.
Bliss Lau, p. 127, Matthew Brookes.
Bliss Lau Bodychains, p. 128-133, Billy Kidd (photos),